Inscribed for my esteemed
colleague and long time friend,
Willard L. Marmelzat,
with best wishes,
Richard L. Sutton Jr.

SIXTEENTH CENTURY PHYSICIAN AND HIS METHODS

MERCURIALIS ON DISEASES OF THE SKIN

HIC LIBER
STUDIOSIS MEDICINAE
DEDICATUR

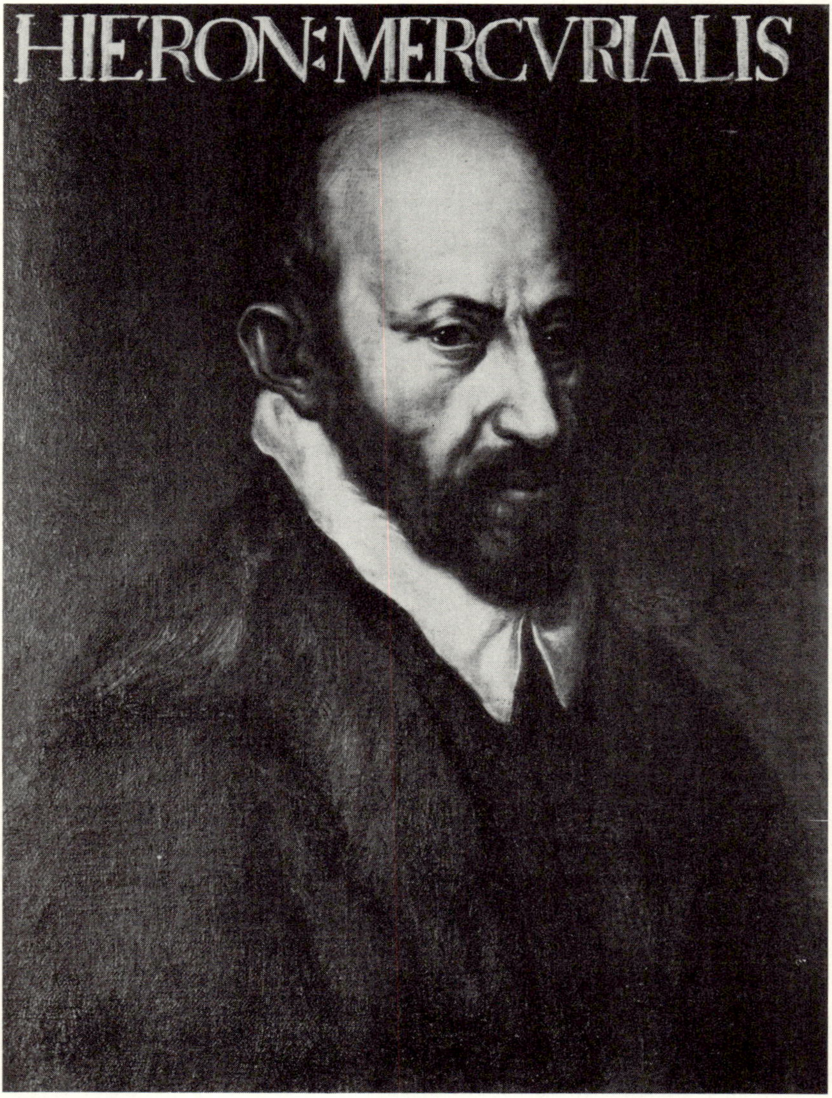

Portrait from the Uffizi Gallery.

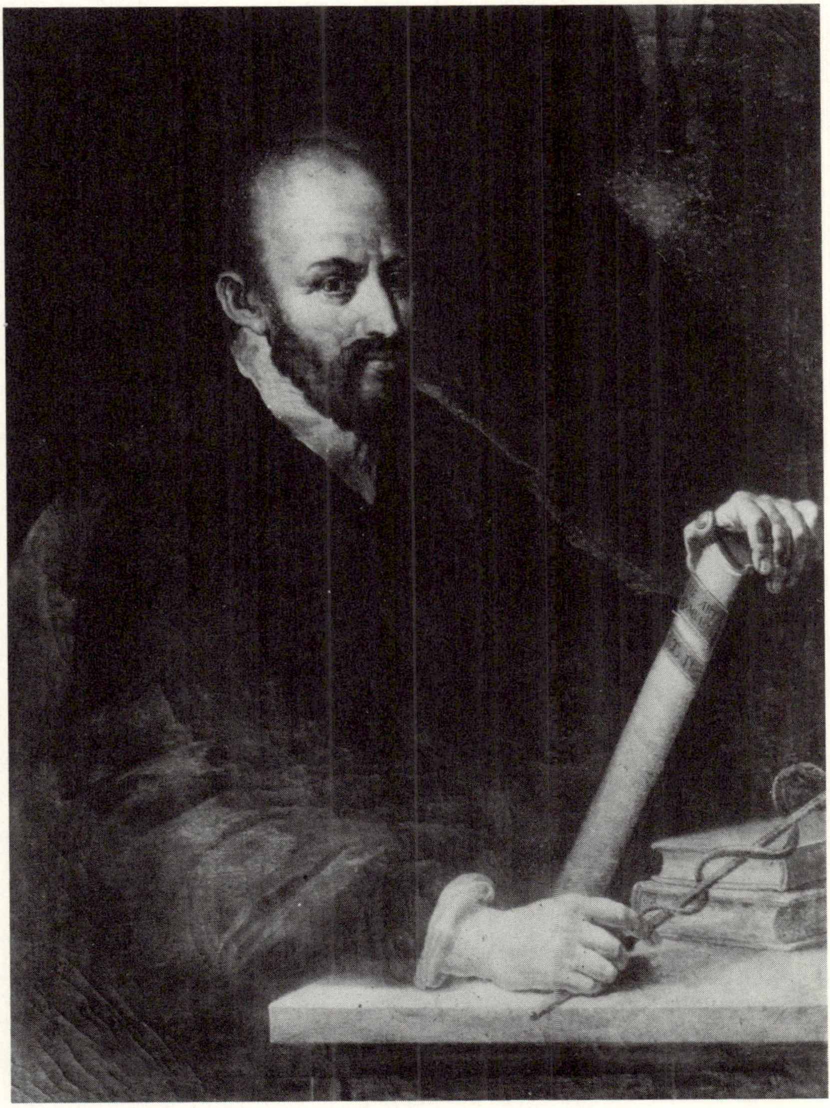

Portrait from Fratelli Alinari.

TWO PORTRAITS OF THE FRONTISPIECE

Left—Portrait provided by the Uffizi Gallery, Florence, Italy, with the comment, "Author unknown." (See Capparoni, 1928; Gior. Ital. D & S 73:1106, 1934.)

Right—Hieronymus Mercurialis (1530-1606), from Fratelli Alinari, Florence, Italy, who knew only that "This painting was photographed by our firm during a 1929 exhibition of portraits of scientists at the Museum of Science in Florence." Dr. Margherita Lenzini of the Gallery expressed the opinion that "Perhaps the painting belongs to Giovio (1483-1552), from which a copy now in our collection was later made." Mercurialis' De Arte Gymnastica, when published in 1569, did not look like the book in the portrait, Dr. Jerome Pierce Webster told me. The painter here shows the second edition, published several years after Mercurialis' death. Dr. Lenzini stated, "It is perhaps correct to suppose a portrait now unknown did exist, from which were taken the portrait in the Giovio Collection and, later, the one with the book. The latter was done by a better artist." Daniel MacMorris, Kansas City portrait painter, observed that the likeness contains detail suggesting that it was painted from life. The book could have been added later.

SIXTEENTH CENTURY PHYSICIAN AND HIS METHODS

MERCURIALIS ON DISEASES OF THE SKIN

THE FIRST BOOK ON THE SUBJECT (1572)

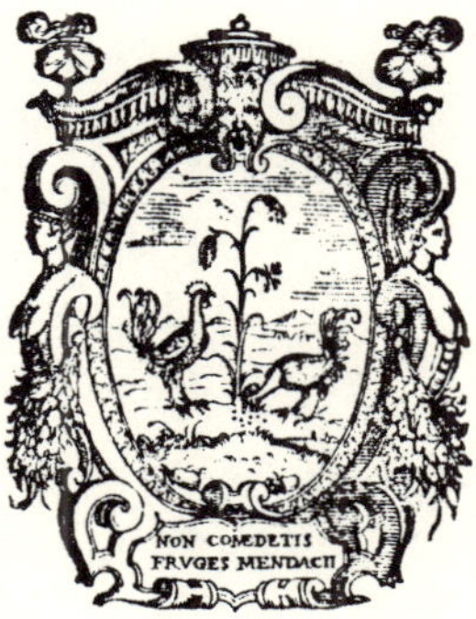

Translation from the Latin, Glossary, and Commentary by

Richard L. Sutton, Jr., MD, ScD, FRS Edin.

Emeritus Clinical Professor, Dermatology, University of Kansas

Adjunct Professor, Medicine, Ophthalmology, and Geosciences, University of Missouri-Kansas City

Honorary Member of the American Academy of Dermatology and of the American Dermatological Association

THE LOWELL PRESS / KANSAS CITY, MISSOURI
1986

First Edition

Library of Congress Catalog Card Number 85-82669
ISBN 0-932845-12-6

Printed in the United States of America
by The Lowell Press of Kansas City

Books are available at $37.50 per copy
from the author
3203 West 83rd Terrace, Leawood, Kansas 66206
and from The Lowell Press Inc.
115 East 31st Street, P.O. Box 1877, Kansas City, Missouri 64141

CONTENTS

FOREWORD

THE CATALOGUE of old books offered, "Mercuriali, Geronimo: De Morbis Cutaneis et Omnibus Corporis Humani Excrementis Tractatus. Small 4to, old vellum (old repairs to margins of first 4 leaves). Venice, apud P. & A. Meietos, 1572. First Edition . . . The first systematic text-book on diseases of the skin according to Garrison-Morton 3980."

De Morbis Cutaneis—On Diseases of the Skin—1572! Irresistible, any history of medicine enthusiast or dermatologist would agree, especially a dermatologist who has written, revised, or contributed to a book so titled. At the time this text, four hundred years old, came into my possession, I had published ten such books (see Sutton, 1981).

My need to know who Mercurialis was, and what he thought, and how he thought, was not to be withstood. My Latin was the residue of four years of secondary school exposure that ended in 1923. So I assembled, and over a period of time exploited, a considerable number of friends, strangers, dictionaries, and reference books, and put together in English typescript a biography of Mercurialis, a translation of his book, a glossary in which all the things and all the proper names he mentioned were identified, all the portraits and engravings of the man ever published, and a bibliography as complete as I could make it.

The extraordinary help of certain individuals requires acknowledgment.

The Reverend Richard Daniel Brigham, Episcopal priest, was at that time a college undergraduate who was—and is, of course—far more interested in old books and ancient languages than in sports or jalopies. The enthusiastic collaboration of the younger man and the older is a delightful memory. For us, the task was long and difficult. Of interest was the usefulness of my medical sophistication. When the Latin-English dictionaries offered alternatives, it was easy for me to choose the word that made sense. The sixteenth century doctor and I thought a good deal alike.

Irene Blase, retired from a long career of teaching Latin in the

Kansas City, Missouri, School District, was extremely competent. If I were speaking instead of writing, I would expatiate on her excellences. When this petite maiden lady died at age 90 in 1985, I lost a dear friend.

Prof. Coleman H. Benedict must be mentioned with some detail. He was a classicist of Columbia University, New York, New York, upon whose kindness Dan and I imposed when the words or rhetoric baffled us. We would beg him for help, and in the disciplined hand of the elderly scholar not provided with a secretary, he would reply that he was immensely overburdened but would accommodate us just this once. We succeeded in persuading him to do so several times, and we wrote him the most gracious thank-you notes we could compose, with the intent to impose on him further. One of the dead ends from which he extricated us was when the Latin, not punctuated in the sixteenth century, tail-spun in a direct quotation as indecipherable to us as Sumerian.

Adolph Rostenberg, Jr., M.D., of Chicago, gave the formal discussion of the paper on Mercurialis that I read before the American Dermatological Association in 1966, published in the A.M.A. *Archives of Dermatology* 94:763-772 (Dec.) 1966. With permission, I republish much of this essay in the Introduction. Dr. Rostenberg kindly approved my reprinting his discussion, which exemplifies, as have his publications and spoken words for many years, his scholarship, resourcefulness, independence of thought, and artistry in articulation, characteristics greatly appreciated by his contemporaries.

Mrs. Marguerite Brown, of Raytown, Missouri, was patient and precise in her secretarial work of transforming my copy into typescript. She reads my handwriting easily, she says.

Overcoming with difficulty my fondness for anecdotes, I list others to whom I am especially indebted.

Harry Arnold, Jr., M.D., whose editorial eye caught a number of slips in the typescript and whose patience in finding these represents gracious friendship;

Mrs. James R. Blacker (Mrs. Brigham's mother) and Mrs. Richard Daniel Brigham, whose encouragement and secretarial assistance were invaluable to Dan Brigham and me;

John B. Blake, Ph.D., Chief, History of Medicine Division, National Library of Medicine, Bethesda, Maryland, who located many biographic references;

Lydia Bowen, Librarian, County of Los Angeles, Department of Arboreta and Botanical Gardens, Arcadia, California, who identified numerous herbs and provided descriptions of them;

George Bryde, Associate Professor of Philosophy, Avila College, Kansas City, Missouri, whose Greek scholarship was extremely helpful;

Roy F. Butler, Ph.D., Department of Classics, Baylor University, Waco, Texas, whose advice on several topics was much appreciated;

Cecil C. Coad, A.B., former head of the History Department, Pembroke-Country Day School, Kansas City, Missouri, who at my request prepared a historical perspective of the sixteenth century;

Archibald M. H. Cray, K.C.V.O., of London, an inspiring senior dermatologist, who loaned me his 1625 edition of Mercurialis' *De Morbis Cutaneis;*

Mansour Ali Haseeb, Dean, Faculty of Medicine, University of Khartoum, Republic of the Sudan, who answered a number of queries concerned with early Arabic medical scholars;

Miss Jean Husted, of the editorial offices of the Dorland Medical Dictionaries, W. B. Saunders Co., Philadelphia, who identified many words of both Latin and Greek derivation and clarified their etymology;

Mrs. George E. Lehr, my secretary prior to my retirement in 1976;

Mrs. Jill Maidhof, my reader, whose cheerful and intelligent help and 20/20 vision in effect made the enterprise possible;

Ralph H. Major, M.D., Professor Emeritus of Medicine and of History of Medicine, University of Kansas Medical Center, who, with the late Logan Clendening, M.D., deserves great credit for the excellence of the History of Medicine collection, and who, with the publisher, was gracious with permission to quote from his *History of Medicine,* Charles C Thomas, Publisher, Springfield, Illinois, 1954;

Phoebe Peck, History of Medicine Librarian, Clendening Medical Library, University of Kansas Medical Center, who seemed able to find anything;

Edward Sintz, Head, Social Sciences Department, and the members of his staff, Kansas City, Missouri, Public Library.

A gentleman whose anonymity I will preserve was inspirational in his way. A professor in a local college, he replied to my query as to the meaning of the abbreviation "S.D." that I ought to give up the project. In a roundabout way I learned that "S.D." which appears early in the text at the top of a dedicatory preface by Aicardius, means "Salutem Dictu," or, roughly, "Salutations having been given," or "Dear Sir." Once learned, this stays in an average memory. My mother, whose maiden name was Magdalena Schüssler Igel, was of pure German lineage, and my fifty percent provided the stubbornness that carried me through. May all the students of that professor remember him as gratefully as I do.

In translation, the liberties I felt obliged to take were especially in devising English acceptable to my contemporaries, who are accustomed to text from which disposable words have been disposed of, and the reader's life span is treated as if it were valuable. Renaissance Latin is not self-conscious when it uses two words, or sentences, where one would do, and it is not monosyllabic. Aicardius' Latin double negatives and perpetual passive voice were annoying. I used English. When structure was overlapping and repetitive, I condensed. The redundance if translated literally would be intolerable. A specimen occurs in Alexander's argument as to why the feet are less subject to pigmentary abnormalities than the hands (Book 2, Chapter 2). In such morasses, I felt that I was trying to make crisp prints from out-of-focus negatives.

The text is Aicardius' transcription of Mercurialis' lectures, not of his writing, and I presumed some of the prerogatives of a re-write editor. The words I have used, as seldom seen today as some of them are, appear in Webster (1938).

The glossary, fascinating to me, and I hope to others, explains many of them and highlights the intellectual background of their use. In many instances it indicates their etymology. It identifies proper names as well as unfamiliar concepts and things. It is filled with "quaint and curious lore" and the direct quotations of charming antique English.

Occasionally words that might require reference to a glossary are defined parenthetically in situ to save the reader's time.

Dan Brigham prepared much of the literal translation. Mercurialis lectured, his lectures were transcribed by his student, Aicardius, and Aicardius' Latin flowed through our minds, doubtless with some eddies and backwashes, conceivably picking up a bit of foreign material despite our caution.

In offering a free rendition of the original, I tried to avoid altering

Mercurialis' meaning, as Aicardius in his preface says he too tried to do. I sought to avoid arrogation of what is contemporary, trying not to give Mercurialis more credit than is his due. His views prove often consistent with our own, although grounded on what is to a great extent obsolete, from our point of vantage.

As the work of translation proceeded, my curiosity was supplanted by a fascination that will prove contagious, I hope, to others, whose imagination may be caught up with the vivid reality of the days of old, the practice and science of medicine, the pharmacopea then available, the judgment and resourcefulness of the physician, and his concern for the interests of the patient that has characterized medicine throughout history. The scholarship, the personalities of Mercurialis and of the authors he quoted from Hippocrates to Cornarius (d. ca 1566), the bringing to life of these people, their wisdom, their occasional errors, their disputations—insight into all this lies in and between the lines.

Mercurialis' 16 lectures, while uneven in length, averaged perhaps 3,000 words, a feasible quantity to present in one lecture. Thus he offered his students more than present-day curriculum committees are likely to permit a dermatologist to give. His presentations are professionally didactic and practical. He followed traditional medical description, giving nomenclature, historical resumés, etiology, symptomatology, and treatment.

That Mercurialis was a great teacher and practitioner is evident. His concern for his patients is apparent in many passages. He noted the effect of anger on pruritus. In this book he made no mention of acne or of contact dermatitis, unless "dew" was a cause, but in his *De Decoratione* there is much dermatology not found here.

His materia medica contained more items than mine. His medicinals are as obscure to me as penicillin would be to him, but we have the advantage, for we were born later. To find out what he thought and what he prescribed and why are main interests of this essay. The glossary is informative.

Two Latin dictionaries were constantly at hand: that edited by F. Leverett, *A New and Copious Lexicon of the Latin Language,* compiled chiefly from *The Magnum Totius Latinitatis Lexicon of Fucciolati and Forcellini and the German works of Scheller and Leunemann,* Boston, J. M. Wilkins and R. B. Carter and C. C. Little and James Brown, 1841; and that of Carlton T. Lewis and Charles Short, *A Latin Dictionary, founded on Andrews' Edition of Freund's*

Latin Dictionary, Oxford University Press, 1879 (impression of 1962).

The Webster's dictionaries, accredited in the bibliography of the glossary, especially those of 1918 and 1938, are remarkably informative. The lists include almost every word I needed, many of which are obsolete. Many obscure New Latin words when anglicized turned up in Webster.

When a Latin word did not go into English satisfactorily, I used an approximation and put the Latin word in parentheses following, or vice versa.

Finding the meanings of some words was like hunting Easter eggs. The word "tyria," for example, was tantalizing. Nothing under "T" in any reference book I tried. In a moment of inspiration, I listened to the word instead of looking at it. "Phthirus"—louse—of course, as any dermatologist ought to have figured out.

Sixteenth century Latin sentences were sparingly punctuated. Only one em separated a period from the next letter, which might or might not be capitalized. Quotation marks would not be used for at least another century. While the Latin was run in without paragraphing, I paragraphed where it seemed to be a good idea.

The Latin pages of the 1572 book are numbered at the end of the running head on the right. The right leaf carries a running head that reads either "Liber Primus" or "Liber Secundus," and the left, "De Morbis Cutaneis." Fifty-two such pages contain the treatise on the skin.

Illustrative material was gathered from every source I could locate, and all I found are incorporated in the book. A doubtful one is the representation published by A. Simili (1942). This so differs from the others that I wonder if it is correctly identified.

The reality of the distant past is almost as difficult to apprehend as that of the future, for one has experienced neither. A hundred years seems comprehensible to me when I think of the interval between the birth of my father and the marriage of my first grandchild. This is a unit of time I can grasp and fill in with a myriad of details. Four such units ago, Hieronymus Mercurialis (1530-1606) ate and slept, was surrounded by family, friends, and current events, and studied, practiced, and taught medicine.

"Often called the first century of the modern world," wrote Cecil C. Coad, "the sixteenth was one of action in all areas of endeavor. The Renaissance had reached its maturity. The old masters,

Leonardo da Vinci (d. 1519), Raphael (d. 1520), and Michael Angelo (d. 1540) had lived well into the century, and new masters were appearing who were concerned with human problems and observational science. That Joshua commanded the sun to stand still was no longer proof that the rotation of the earth is not responsible for night and day. Erasmus, Copernicus, Cervantes, Galileo, Kepler, Shakespeare, and a host of others evidenced the change in thinking. Human beings, as well as divine, challenged attention. One's self as well as one's soul was an object of concern. Ignorance and superstition were being replaced by inquiry and experiment, and the tremendous increase of knowledge was evident.

"Discovery and exploration of the New World stirred the imagination as it had not been stirred for centuries. Vast amounts of gold and silver from the New World (much of it stolen by conquest) were pouring into Europe, where a shortage had existed for a thousand years, a shortage which was one of the causes of the downfall of the Roman Empire in the west. The discovery of an all-water route to India (1498) led to enormous expansion of trade and the shifting of the commercial world from the Mediterranean to the Atlantic, with conspicuous effects on western states, Portugal, Spain, and the Netherlands at first but eventually on all the countries of western Europe.

"The Reformation was the great movement of the century, and it profoundly influenced other great changes. The posting of Luther's Ninety-five Theses was a dramatic incident in the movement born of inquiry and the search for truth, but Luther was not the first, nor was he alone. Erasmus, Zwingli, Colet, More, Calvin, and others were leaders in the examination of religious problems. The result was a Counter-Reformation within the Church itself and a cleavage in Christendom that left the northern part of Europe and England Protestant, while southern Europe and the countries nearer Rome remained Catholic.

"Spain became the great Defender of the Faith, and this, along with the insult to the Spanish royal family by the divorce in 1533 of Catherine of Aragon by Henry VIII, led to conflict with England that was terminated by the defeat of the Great Armada, to Spain a fateful event indeed, and to England a boon. In the meantime Spain, under the impact of her new-found wealth in America, and influenced by her long proximity to the advanced civilization of the Moors, was enjoying her Golden Age. Mohammedan culture, particularly in science, mathematics, medicine, and architecture, had extended its influence to some degree over all of Europe, notably after the fall of Constantinople in 1453, but its influence was greatest in Spain, where the Mohammedans had been entrenched since 711 A.D.

"The break from the authority of the Church incident to the Reformation gave people, both in Germany and elsewhere, the temerity to doubt and challenge authorities in the political, economic, and social orders. The revolution in the minds of men was clearly reflected in all aspects of the history of those times. It was this great century that provided the atmosphere of the life and work of Hieronymus Mercurialis."

Illuminating, I believe, are the prefatory paragraphs of Arturo Castiglioni, whom I quote with permission from "The Life and Times of Gaspare Tagliacozzi, Surgeon of Bologna, 1545-1599, With a Documented Study of the Scientific and Cultural Life of Bologna in the Sixteenth Century," by Martha Gnudi and Jerome Pierce Webster, published by Herbert Reichner, New York (1950).

"Among the most distinguished physicians of the Renaissance there tower the figures of three great masters: Jacopo Berengario da Carpi, Andreas Vesalius, and Gaspare Tagliacozzi. These men, though still bound by scholastic tradition, felt the impact of the new currents of thought and action that flowed through the universities with the rebirth of literature and art, and themselves opened new pathways in the evolution of medical studies. All three were at once both anatomists and surgeons in an era when anatomy was still taught according to the text of Galen and when anatomical dissections were performed but infrequently. At Bologna and Padua the necessity for personal observation founded on dissection had already been recognized, and this formed the basis of regular anatomical teaching. At a time when surgery had no place in medical schools throughout the rest of Europe and when bitter controversies raged between physicians and surgeons, at Bologna and Padua anatomy and surgery were already taught by the same university professor, so firmly accepted was the concept that the two disciplines are closely bound together.

"Jacopo Berengario da Carpi (1470-1530), precursor of Vesalius in anatomical research, daring in his surgical procedures, and expert in diagnosis, was the first Italian anatomist of this epoch. Andreas Vesalius (1514-1564), who brought to Padua his inexhaustible passion for anatomical studies pursued by an expert surgeon, victoriously led the way to scientific anatomy freed of Galenic limitations. Gaspare Tagliacozzi (1545-1600), eminent anatomist and surgeon, pupil and successor of Giulio Cesare Aranzio in the chair of anatomy at Bologna, was the first to describe in detail, and to practice with admirable skill and sure ability, that branch of surgery which today we call plastic surgery.

"These great masters were, in every aspect of their multiple activities, truly men of their times. Animated by the passion for study and a thirst for glory, fully aware of their own potentialities and of the importance of their work, they were profoundly influenced by the cultured atmosphere in which they lived. The brilliant rebirth of Italian art—which not only dominated painters and sculptors but also exercised its fecund and penetrating influence on the philosopher and the physician alike, on the artisan, the merchant, and the man of public affairs—is manifest also in the work of these illustrious physicians."

To these masters, I would add the encyclopedic scholar, Hieronymus Mercurialis. His field was medicine, not surgery. He was less original, less aggressive, and more erudite.

DE MORBIS CVTANEIS ET OMNIBVS CORPORIS HVMANI EXCREMENTIS

TRACTATVS

locupletiſsimi, uariaq́ue doctrina referti, non ſolum Medicis, uerum etiam Philoſophis magnopere utiles,

Ex ore HIERONYMI MERCVRIALIS Medici clariſsimi diligenter excepti, atque in Libros Quinque digeſti.

OPERA PAVLI AICARDII.

CVM LICENTIA, ET PRIVILEGIO,

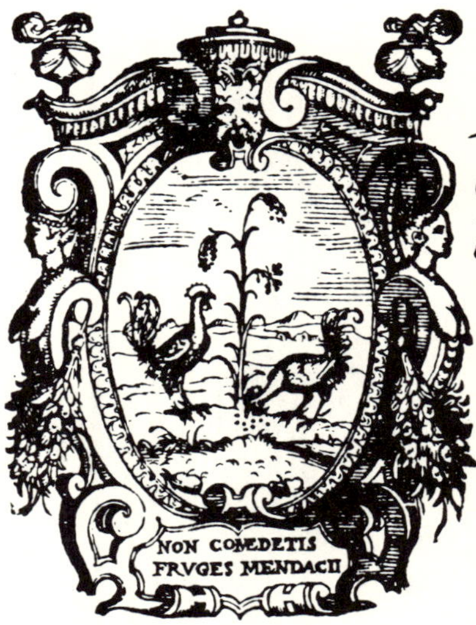

Ex librij
Joseph
Graffagnino
Calatrb. E

VENETIIS,

Apud Paulum, & Antonium Meietos fratres Bibliopo' Patauinos. M. D. LXXII.

INTRODUCTION

THE TITLE PAGE reads as follows. On Diseases of the Skin and All Excrements of the Human Body, with copious references to numerous and diverse doctrines, useful not only to physicians but also to philosophers, carefully compiled from the words of the most illustrious physician, Hieronymus Mercurialis, and arranged in five books by Paulus Aicardius, with authorization and approval. Venice, Paulus and Antonius Meietus Brothers, Publishers, 1572.

The motto within the publishers' emblem reads, "Swallow not the fruit of error."

Richard Daniel Brigham and I, with the assistance of many consultants, as noted in the Foreword, translated the portion of this book on diseases of the skin. I edited it and provided the glossary and illustrations.

Mercurialis lectured 400 years ago. His lectures were transcribed by his student, Paulus Aicardius, who published *De Morbis Cutaneis. . . .*

Our literal translation needed emendation provided by familiarity with medicine, and I employed such English as I judged might be read with pleasure.

In Forli, Italy, Camilla Pungectori bore a son to Johannus Mercurialis on the day sacred to the memory of St. Jerome (Hieronymus Sophronius Eusebius, about 340 to 420), whose name they gave their infant. The family was an old one of good reputation but not of noble lineage.

As a young man, Hieronymus Mercurialis was educated in Greek and philosophy, studied medicine at Padua, and returned to Forli to practice, "giving equal attention to curing the sick and expounding the books of Greek philosophers and medical men" (Boerner, 1755). His prominence and scholarly repute were such that his fellow citizens sent him as a delegate to Pope Pius IV in Rome, where he was received by Cardinal Alexander Farnesius. Because of his erudition, eloquence, and personality, he enjoyed the company of the most eminent men of letters, including

This illustration, photographed from the original, was provided by Dr. Walter Vichi from the collections in the Forli Institute of Arts and Culture. It was engraved by Jean Sadeler (b. Brussels 1550, d. Venice 1600), as the inscription indicates.

Dated 1590, it is the earliest of the depictions I have located. It was copied, it would appear, mirror imaged, in Boissard and de Bry, 1598.

The inscription, superlatively florid, identifies the likeness as that of Hieronymus Mercurialis, then proceeds as follows. "Hail to that Great Man, favored by Phoebus, unparalleled Phoenix! Hail, Sun-like Aesculapian and celebrated medical writer! From this countenance the world may judge the upright heart, the fame long known among the stars. Philosopher and educator, born 1530, died 1606." (Done in 1590 by Jean Sadeler.)

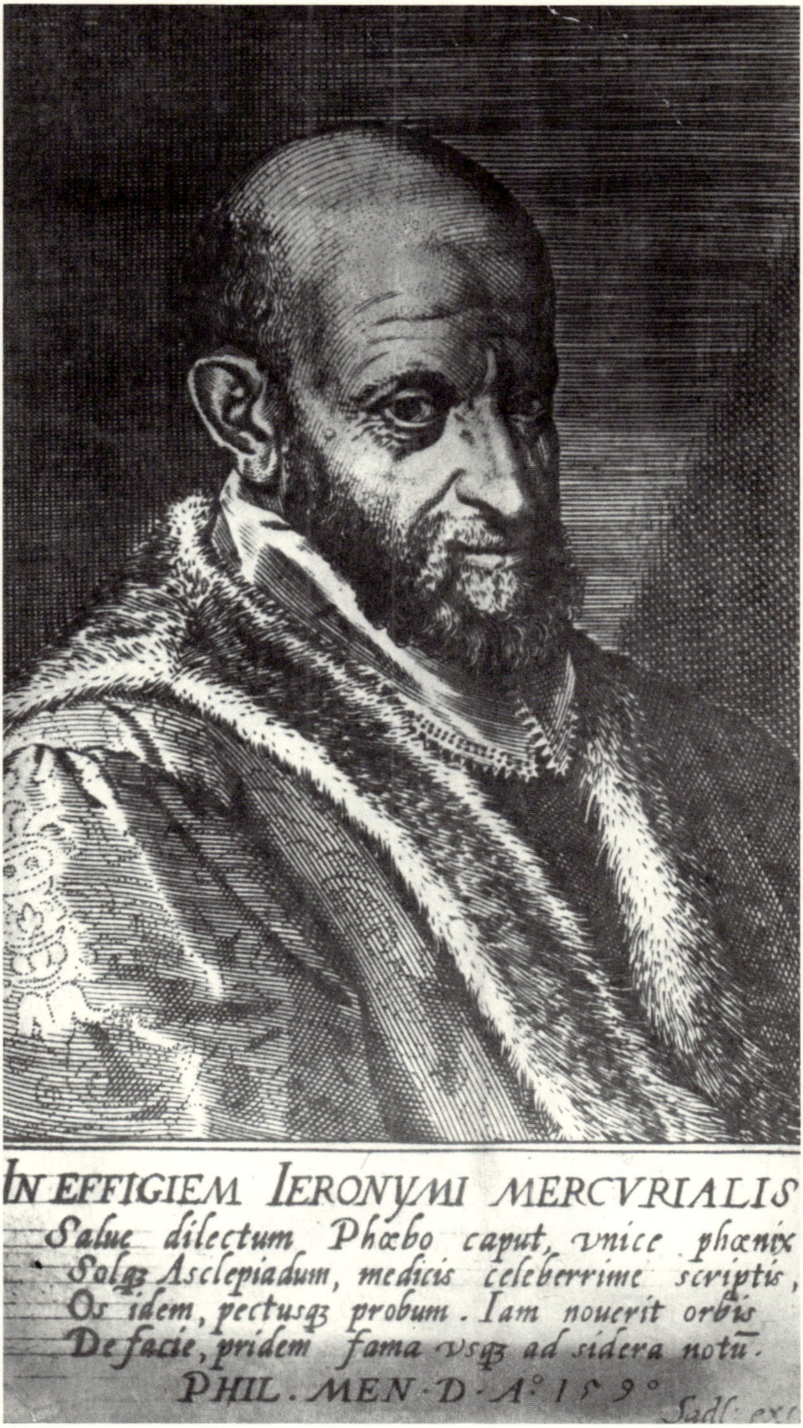
IN EFFIGIEM IERONYMI MERCVRIALIS
Salue dilectum Phœbo caput, vnice phœnix
Solaq; Asclepiadum, medicis celeberrime scriptis,
Os idem, pectusq; probum. Iam nouerit orbis
De facie, pridem fama vsq; ad sidera notū.
PHIL. MEN. D. A°. 1590
Sadl. exc.

This engraving was published in 1598 by Jean Boissard and Theodore de Bry in their Iconographia Virorum Illustrium, Frankfort, 1597-1599, Part 3, page 150. The correct reference was located by Bruce Bradley of Linda Hall Library, Kansas City, Missouri, and the photograph of the engraving was provided by Thomas Lange, of the Huntington Library, San Marino, California.

The engraving dated 1590, in the collections of the Forli Institute of Arts and Culture is notably similar, and the inscription differs only in its condensation as seen here. One may surmise that this is a copy of the earlier one, perhaps having been made by the same artist, Jean Sadeler.

A copper plate copied from it would print as a mirror image, as is seen in Bullart (1682), facsimiles of which were published by Levinson (1929, 1935), Gnudi and Webster (1950), and the author of Medical Greats (1964). Some illustrations appear to have been copies of copies, with the expected loss of detail. The artist is able to print a likeness that is not a mirror image of the subject; but which likeness is not a mirror image cannot be discerned.

Boissard and de Bry's text, pages 151-153, is given in the bibliography.

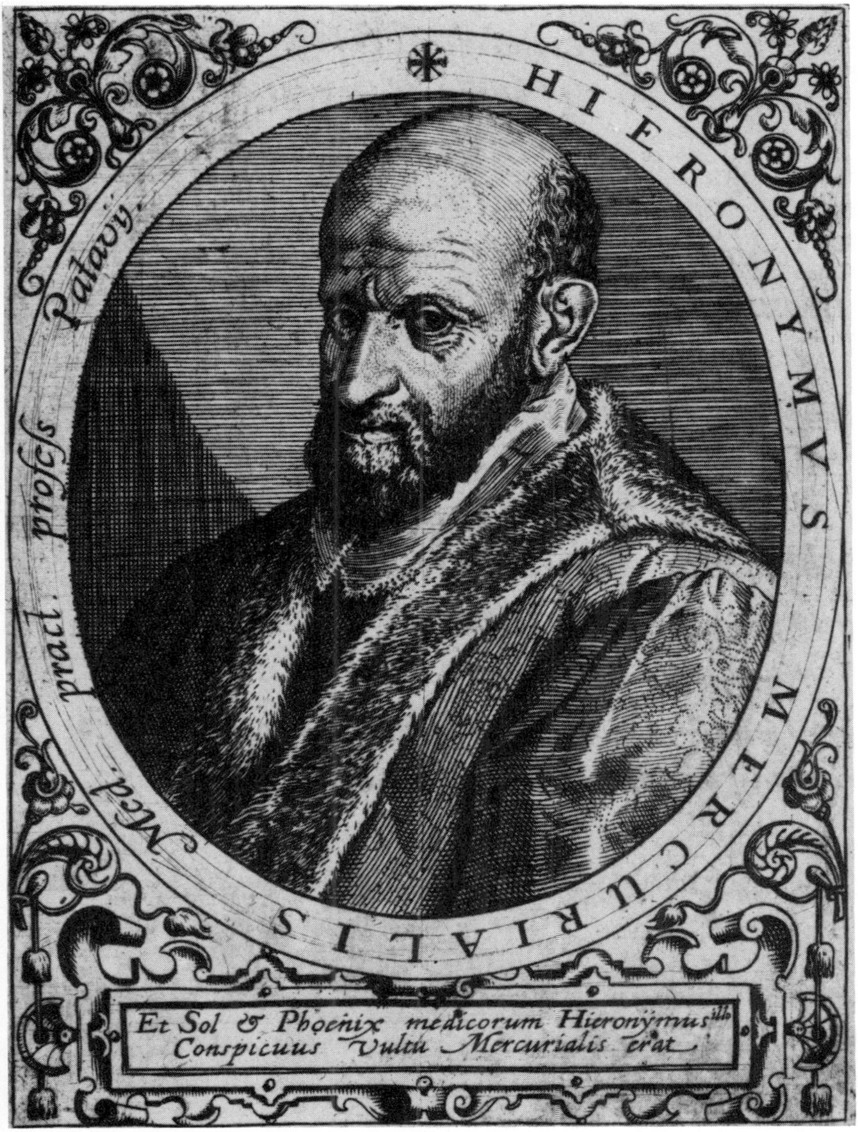
HIERONYMVS MERCVRIALIS
Med. pract. profess. Patavij.
Et Sol & Phoenix medicorum Hieronymus ill
Conspicuus vultu Mercurialis erat

This likeness of Mercurialis appears in Bullart, Acad. d. Sciences . . . *1682, again in Levinson,* Med. Life *36:353, 1929 and 42:344, 1935, and in Gnudi and Webster, 1950, who accredit their illustration to Bullart. It appeared again in the article on Medical Greats, J.A.M.A. 1964.*

Zapf published a mirror image of less detail in 1805. The right cheek is seen in the Sadeler engraving dated 1590, the left cheek in the Boissard and de Bry engraving of 1598. All show the nevus lateral to the eye. Was it on Mercurialis' right or left cheek?

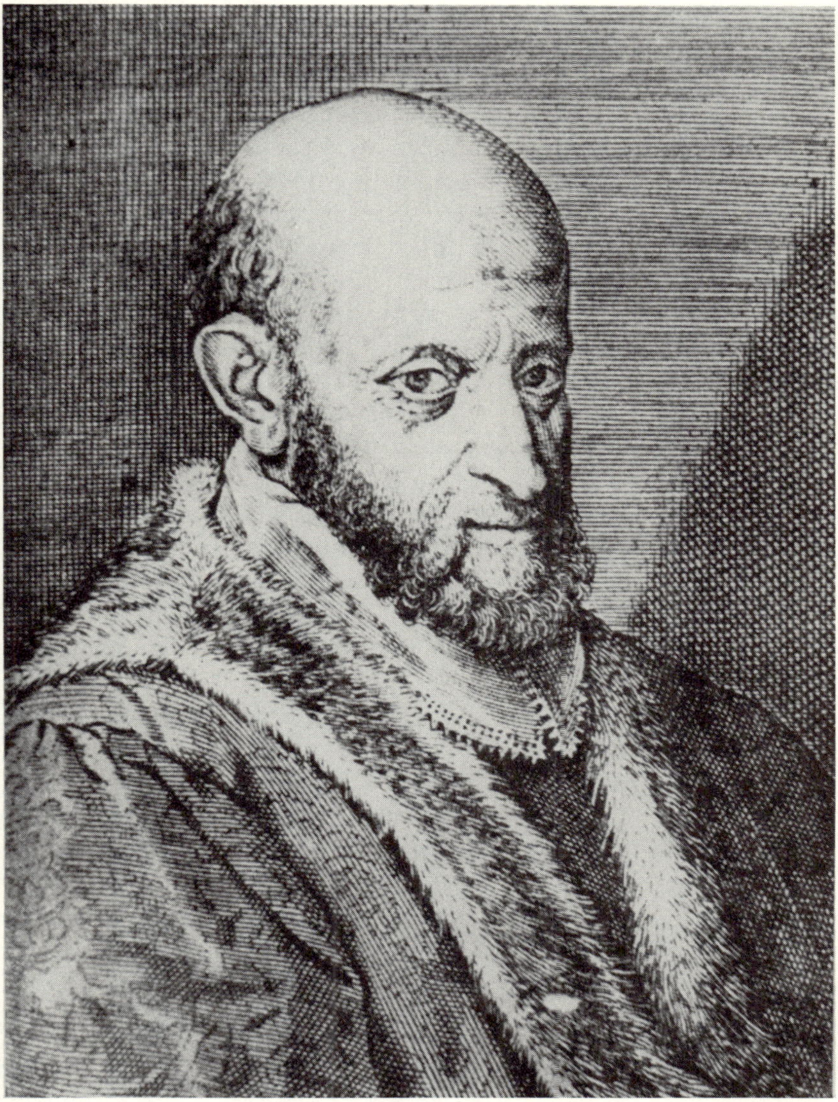

Guglielmo Sirleto, who was the son of a physician, was then a custodian of the Vatican library, and became the Cardinal Sirletus to whom *De Morbis Cutaneis* was dedicated. After seven years in Rome, Mercurialis, having utilized the vast resources of that library, accepted the chair of Medicine at Padua. He attended an illness of the Emperor Maximilian and received distinguished rewards for his services.

I have not located the date of his marriage to Francesca Bici. They named one of their sons Maximilian, after the Emperor. Their other son, Johannes, died in 1597 while he was a student of medicine in Spain. Their beloved and loving daughter was Margherita.

Mercurialis taught at Padua for many years, also at Bologna and Pisa. "He was endowed by a kind nature with a remarkable inborn excellence and a most fortunate disposition, and was assiduously industrious," it was said of him (Boerner, 1775), and "he was decorated with the highest honors in philosophy and medicine, and he behaved very differently from the general run of medical men. Possessed of remarkable skill and of such learning and gentleness of nature, he was in the highest esteem and greatest favor of all good people. For teaching others he seemed born, preferring the peace of literary pursuits and academic life to the courts of princes and munificent fees. He was of unusual comeliness of body, presenting the appearance of a good and honorable man in features and expression, with broad and candid brow and impeccable and pleasing manners. He was an upright man, who lived a life shining with purity and piety."

No other medical writer has single-handedly manifested his astonishing capacity for collating all that was known into specialty texts, many of which were the first of their kind: On the feeding of infants, the art of gymnastics, diseases of the skin, of women, of children, of the eyes, and of the ears, while publishing masses of material on poisons, epidemics, medicines, and the practice of medicine with "the diagnosis and treatment of all diseases of the human body."

I do not provide a critical bibliography of Mercurialis' writings, but I list the titles of his major achievements, in English, arranged chronologically, following Boerner (1775) and Panckoucke (1824). These indicate the scope of his classical knowledge and productivity.

THE MAJOR WORKS OF HIERONYMUS MERCURIALIS

1552 Nomothesaurus, or the care of nursing infants, Padua
1569 The Art of Gymnastics, Venice (one of his most famous; many editions and translations: "The Cradle of Modern Orthopedics")
1570 Various lectures, and the letter of Alexander of Tralles on intestinal worms, Venice
1572 Diseases of the Skin and All Excrements of the Human Body, Venice
1577 Lectures on the plague, Venice
1582 Diseases of Women, Basle
1583 Diseases of Children, Venice (of high repute among pediatricians, with interesting notes on stammering)
1584 On Poisons and Diseases Due to Poisons, Frankfort
1585 A Critique and Arrangement of the Works of Hippocrates, Venice
1588 All Existing Works of Hippocrates of Cos, Venice (a critical collation and restitution of the old codices, rearrangement of the texts, and their translation from Greek to Latin)
1590 On the Composition of Medicines, Venice
1591 Diseases of the Eyes and Ears, Frankfort
1601 Medical practice: The Differential Diagnosis and Treatment of All Affections of the Human Body and an Inquiry into Their Causes, Frankfort

His familiarity with the authorities of the two thousand years from Hippocrates to his contemporaries was such that in Aicardius' preface he said, "They seemed to come alive. He enabled anyone to become confidently intimate with all the Greek, Latin, and Arabic writers."

Such scholarship, including as it did, his translation of all the works of Hippocrates, resulted in his recognition, according to Bellini (1976) as an authoritative Greek philologist.

Mercurialis mentioned the following individuals in *De Morbis Cutaneis,* some of them many times. The medical authorities to whom he referred are marked with asterisks. Dates not designated B.C. are A.D. Indicators are "ca" for "approximately" and "fl" for "flourished," and "?" means the identification is dubious.

*Actuarius	fl ca 1250
Aeschines	ca 389-314 B.C.
*Aesculapius	ca 1200 B.C.
*Aetius	502-575
*Albertus Magnus	1193-1280

*Alexander of Tralles	525-605
Alkman the Poet	fl ca 670 B.C.
*Andromachus (the Younger)	fl 60
*Apollonius	fl ca 180-160 B.C.
*Apponensis (Peter of Abano)	ca 1250-1316
*Appuleius	ca 400
*Archigenes	fl ca 75
*Aristotle	384-322 B.C.
Arrianus	ca 100-170
*Athenaeus	fl ca 50
*Avenzoar	ca 1091-1162
*Averroes	1126-1198
*Avicenna	980-1037
*Cassius	fl 130
*Celsus	ca 25 B.C.-50
*Claudian	fl ca 160
Columella	fl ca 50
*Cornarius	ca 1467-1566
*Crito	ca 100
*Ctesias of Cnidos	ca 400 B.C.
*Dioscorides	440-490
*Empedocles	504-443 B.C.
*Erotianus	ca 50
Festus	?ca 175
Ficinus	ca 1500
*Galen	130-?200
*Guido de Cauliaco (Guy de Chauliac)	ca 1300-1368
*Haly Abbas	ca 930-994
*Hamech ? Father of Mesue	?ca 750
*Heracles of Tarantum	160-110 B.C.
Heroditus	ca 484-425 B.C.
*Hippocrates	?460-377 B.C.
Homer	ca 1100 B.C.
*Jacobus	?ca 460
*Johannitius	809-873
John the Grammarian	ca 600 B.C.
Laitus	?
Leonellus Pius	?
Lucillius Junior	ca 65
*Marcellus	ca 400
*Mesue (Senior)	777-857

*Moses, Rabbi (Maimonides)	1135-1208
*Micander	ca 275 B.C.
*Nicolaus Alexandrinus	?
*Nicolaus Florentinus	ca 1400
*Nicolaus Myrepsos	ca 1250
*Oribasius	fl ca 350
*Pacchius	fl ca 50
*Paulus of Aegina	625-690
Perusinus	ca 25
Pherecydes of Syros	ca 550 B.C.
Plato	428-348 B.C.
Pliny (the Elder)	23-79
*Plotinus	?205-270
Plutarch	ca 46-120
Pollux, Julius	fl ca 150
*Priscianus	fl ca 400
*Protarchus	ca 250 B.C.
*Rhazes	ca 841-926
*Rufus of Ephesus	fl 100
*Serapion	fl ca 900
Serenus, Quintus	fl ca 220
*Soranus of Ephesus	fl ca 98-138
Strabo	ca 64 B.C.-19
Synesius	ca 370-414
*Tagautius	ca 1500-1545
*Theophrastus	370-285 B.C.
*William the Surgeon	ca 1200-1280

I omit details of the bibliographic references that Mercurialis gave within the textual matter. His bibliography was exhaustive, including all who wrote on the subjects from Hippocrates on. Whoever would check his sources will find them in available copies of Mercurialis' original text. Such readers will presumably suffer no language barrier. The chapter and verse footnote citations of Mercurialis' myriad of quotations, the academician's delight, I omit to avoid tediousness of both translating and translation. I would hold readers whom pedantry bores.

The 52 double-pages of *De Morbis Cutaneis* are translated here, but not the 65 pages of *De Excrementis,* which has been largely neglected for 400 years. Irene Blase and I published "Tears" in the *International Journal of Dermatology* of June, 1979. I have Miss

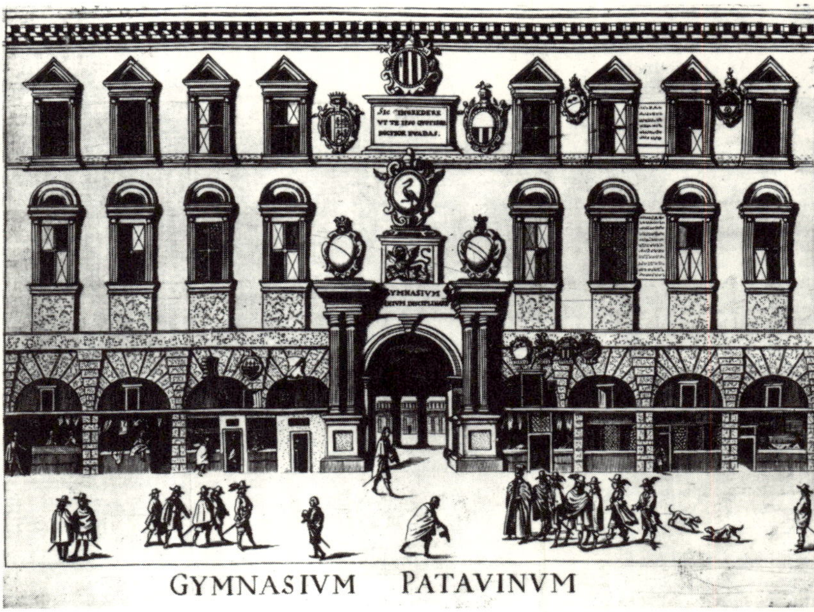

The Gymnasium at Padua, where Mercurialis taught, from an illustration in J. Thomasinus: Gymnasium Paravinus, Utini, Nicolae Schiratti, 1654. The inscription above the entrance reads, "Enter here so that you may yourself someday go forth a teacher." This illustration was used by M. Gnudi and J. P. Webster (1950) in "Tagliacozzi."

Blase's rough literal translations of the other essays and expect to give them to the Kansas University History of Medicine Library. More work than I am able to do is necessary for their publication.

De Excrementis starts with a first book in nine chapters on the urine through page 76 and continues with a second book on the feces in nine chapters, through page 93. A third book contains five chapters, on sweat, pages 94 to 103; tears, pages 103 to 108; sputum, pages 108 to 113; mucus, pages 113 to 115; and discharges from the ears, pages 115 to 117.

In 1623, seventeen years after Mercurialis' death, a volume was published that contained *De Morbis Cutaneis* and several other books for which his lectures had provided the material. Its title page reads as follows:

"Hieronymus Mercurialis, of Forli, the most celebrated and

preeminent physician of his day: Various texts on medical subjects taken accurately from his lectures are here collected and published together after his death, by his grateful medical students.

1. On diseases of women
2. On diseases of children, along with the letter of Trallianus on worms, and verses of other authors; and also on poisons and his notes on poisons.
3. On the plague, from lectures given at Venice and Padua.
4. On diseases of the skin, summarized in three books (sic).
5. On excrements, divided into three books

Lugdunum (Lyons), 1623. Edited by Antonius Pillehotte."

Differences were apparent between the 1572 and 1623 texts of *De Morbis Cutaneis,* but I found no significant additions or deletions. The page size is larger in the 1623 work, and the right and left pages are both numbered. With pages about half again the area of the 1572 text, the 1623 ran 79 pages as compared with 52. The errata listed in the 1572 edition (there were many of them) were corrected. A period was followed by a space and a capital letter, although there continued to be no paragraphing. Chapters were not started on new pages. Prescriptions were tabulated rather than run in, making them much easier to read. Most of the previously abbreviated material was spelled out. In reference to differences between lepra and scabies, on p. 49 left side, the 1572 text reads "magnum," big, while the 1623 text reads "nigram," evil or dire.

Mercurialis' *De Decoratione Liber* edited by Julius Mancino and first published (Panckoucke, 1824) in Frankfort in 1578, contains 88 pages in the 1601 edition published in Venice by Juntas. In it is much material of dermatological interest, on beauty and the lack of it, facial blemishes, the care of the skin and hair, scars, bruises, body odor, wrinkles, warts, calluses, varices, furuncles, sycosis, diseases of the nails, paronychia, and even bad breath.

In *De Morbis Cutaneis,* one must remember that the elements Mercurialis knew were earth, air, fire, and water, and the humors that controlled the constitution were blood, choler, melancholy, and phlegm (see glossary). The materia medica of the medical botanist, Dioscorides (about 40 to 90 A.D., a Greek surgeon in the Roman army of Nero), was augmented but not much altered in fifteen centuries, as evidenced by the *Pharmacopoeia Londònensis* of 1608 (Major, 1954) with substances learned from, for example, *The Royal Book of Haly Abbas* and *The Canon of Avicenna,* those Arabic authors of magnificent achievement of 600 to 700 years previously.

To exemplify Mercurialis' style and views, I point to *De Morbis Cutaneis,* Book 1, Chapter 7 "On Pediculosis." Many of his words and concepts are ill understood today. The glossary is designed to bridge such gaps. Mercurialis' text follows.

"There are some diseases of the scalp with ulceration and others without. The nonulcerative diseases are called 'pediculation' and 'furfuration' (the lousy and the scaly). The ulcerative diseases are achors (small, shallow ulcers) and ceria, or favi, which Aetius and Celsus called 'meliceris' (honeycomb tumors). So we start with the conditions that are not ulcerous and, first, with pediculosis, called by the Greeks 'phthiriasis' (from phtheir, louse). This disease arises from a corruption of the humors and is one in which lice are generated particularly on the head. . . ."

Preparing the glossary gave me an appreciation of the original meanings and etymology of many interesting medical words, some in current use, some obsolete, such as acrochordon (filiform fibroma or wart), alopecia (Greek alopex, fox, a mangy creature), impetigo (Latin verb, attack), mentagra ("the chin disease"), ophiasis (Greek ophis, snake), oxymel (acid—vinegar—and honey), pisseleum (pine tar), pompholyx (bubbly scum of smelted ore), scabies (the scabby disease), treacle (from theriaca, an antidotal cure-all, from Greek ther, venomous animal). The old word for vitriol was chalcanthite, etymologically "flowers of bronze." It was used inexplicitly by some authorities for either green vitriol, ferrous sulfate, or blue vitriol, copper sulfate. Mercurialis tells us,

In the Institute of Arts and Culture in Forli is this bust of Mercurialis done by an unknown sculptor probably of the nineteenth century, according to Dr. Walter Vichi of the Institute.

The inscription on the pedestal reads as follows: Hieronymus Mercurialis of Forli: Because of his proficiency in the Greek language, philosophy, and literature, and because of his remarkable scholarship, this man who for seventeen years exemplified and taught the precepts of medicine in Padua, Bologna, and Pisa, was respected and sought out by the greatest kings of Europe, who, recognizing his eminence, heaped upon him the greatest honors and treasures.

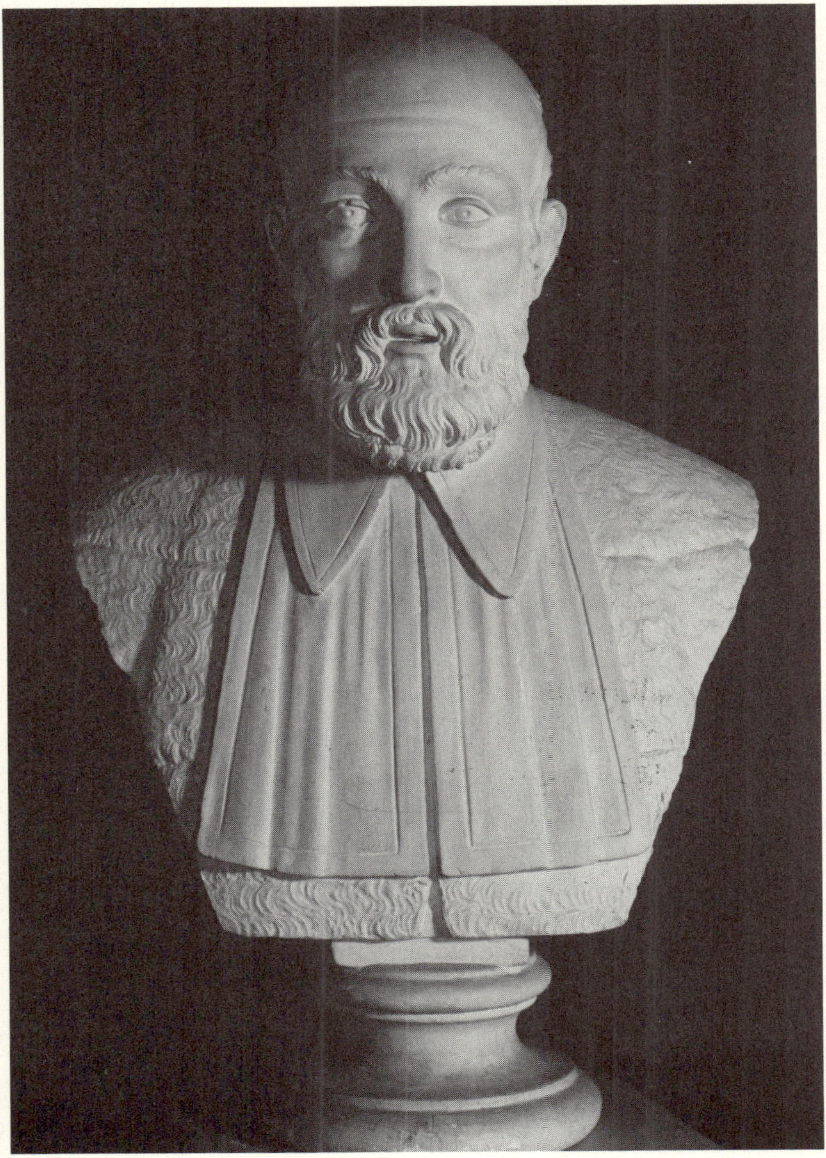

"Rhazes wrote that a friend of his cured graying of the hair by taking a dram of chalcanthite every evening, but Galen damned chalcanthite as an oral medication." One may surmise that some unfortunate Roman with graying hair took blue vitriol and embarrassed his practitioner.

Mercurialis' life ended on November 9, 1606, a life of scholarship, achievement, serenity, and recognition. (See Bett, Brambilla, Capparoni, Cardini, Bellini, Haberling and Vierordt, Simili, Tomasinus, Busacchi et al., and Paoletti.) His terminal illness at the age of 76 was related to the huge kidney stones which he knew he had and which were found at the limited autopsy he had requested. It was said that he met death with equanimity (Boerner). His body was placed in the Abbey of San Mercuriale in Forli in a chapel he and his wife had prepared for their son, Johannus, who died at the age of 25. A marble bust was commissioned for the Forli Museum by his townspeople, who so honored no other physician.

ADOLPH ROSTENBERG, JR., M.D., discussed the paper here excerpted, which I read at the 1966 meeting of the American Dermatological Association:

We are indebted to Dr. Sutton for bringing us a topic off the beaten path. Historical subjects are no longer as popular as once they were; yet, without arguing the merits of this proposition, I believe this is a loss.

Whitehead described European philosophy as a series of footnotes to Plato. I should like to paraphrase this and describe medicine up to 1800 as a series of footnotes to Galen.

Mercurialis, despite the fact that he was one of the great physicians of his day, had views on medicine that clung to the past and were absurd by modern standards. To wit (from *De Morbis Cutaneis*, translated by Dr. Sutton):

"Excrements cannot be supplied when for some reason the brain shrinks, for as long as the brain fills the cranium it moistens the whole skin and maintains its nutrition. If the brain withdraws from the cranium, the skin will want for an abundance of moisture and will be unable to supply the hair with the necessary nutrient. Aristotle said that this may come about through coitus. If indeed the brain declines in people who overindulge, a balding process will quickly follow."

I quote further. "I (Mercurialis) may be asked why nature has not provided man with a pile that is tough and not prone to shedding, and further why, if calvities is injurious to health, should not nature show greater concern for our welfare than for that of beasts?

"I reply as Plato did with regard to the structure of the human head:

nature's plan is that the human head should be designed so as to possess the capability of both bodily health and mental function. If nature wished the head to produce durable hair, man would surely have been incapable of mental activity. Synesius the Philosopher put it cleverly: 'Prudence and pili are incompatible.' Thus the hairiest creatures, sheep for example, are the stupidest (imprudentissima), while those with few hairs, man for example, are the wisest (prudentissima)."

Another absurd belief of the time was the view that by inspection of the urine not only a diagnosis but a prognosis could be made. This practice was so prevalent that physicians are commonly portrayed in Renaissance art as holding a vial of urine. The believers in this practice became known as uromancers, or pisse-prophets. The following is the title page of a book of 1637 condemning these practices. This title page and much other delightful discussion of this subject are given in an article by Dr. Joseph H. Kiefer (Trans. Amer. Assoc. Genitourin. Surg. 50:161-172, 1958).

THE PISSE-PROPHET or
CERTAINE PISSE-POT LECTURES

Wherein are newly discovered the old fallacies, deceit, and jugling of the Pisse-pot Science, used by all those (whether Quacks and Empiricks, or other methodicall Physicians) who pretend knowledge of Diseases, by the Urine, in giving judgement of the same. By Tho. Brian, M.P. lately in the Citie of London, and now in Colchester in Essex.

Never heretofore published by any man in the English Tongue.

Si populus vult decipi, decipiatur.

LONDON.

Printed by E. P. for R. Thrale, and are to be sold at his shop at the signe of the Crosse-Keyes, at Pauls gate.

1637

Dr. Sutton has gone back 400 years, which brings us roughly to the end of the Renaissance. During this period there were outstanding geniuses; yet few important discoveries were made. The fascinating problem is, why did those people think as they did? Not only were certain of their beliefs ludicrous, indeed they were palpably absurd and could easily have been proved to be incorrect; but no attempt was made to test them. Why were no important discoveries made in physics, chemistry, and medicine prior to 1600? Why did they not interrogate, investigate? Why did they not seek the answers by experimentation rather than by explication?

I believe the explanation stems directly from the attitude inculcated by the early Christian Church. In Greek thought knowledge had been a form of virtue, but with the triumph of Christianity this interpretation of experience wavered and fell. The universe became the creation of an inscrutable and suprarational deity that desired not comprehension but worship. Its preeminence depended not on the sovereignty of reason but on the sovereignty of its power. Augustine (quoted in *The Dignity of Man*, Boston: Harvard University Press, 1947), whose thinking dominated the Christian Church for a thousand years, said:

"To seek to limit the inscrutable ways of God by criteria of human reason is to fall into the deep abyss of blasphemy." In his view, contemplation and devotion and submission are man's highest function. The baleful effort to investigate, to question, to come to conclusions on the basis of reason is both useless and impious. Man can know only what God chooses to reveal to him, and His Church is the sole channel and repository of revelation. What God wills must be good because He wills it, not because it is rational. Sovereignty supplants intelligence.

Aquinas attempted to loosen the bonds of reason as demanded by faith. The apparently obvious fact of causation led Aquinas to interpret God as the uncaused cause of everything. He pointed out that the world is a spectacle of incalculable order and harmony. He cited, as examples, so that a man might walk, he has legs; so that a bird might fly, it has wings; so that a wolf might stalk its prey, it has a highly refined capacity for smelling.

This, while allowing man to think, nevertheless circumscribed the arena in which his thoughts could operate. He could think, but only in terms of interpreting an omniscient and beneficent deity that had created everything and necessarily had a good reason for doing so. If only man had the wit to perceive, the reasons would be revealed. Unfortunately, with this approach, there were as many reasons as reasoners.

It was only beginning with Galileo that man attempted to find things out by the experimental method. He tested his abstract world of thought against the dirty, stubborn, and oftentimes unmanageable facts of the real world. It is this attitude that has enabled us to develop our knowledge of material things to the surpassing degree that we have. On the other hand, even today we too often cling to authority and make unsupported assertions. As an example from our own field of dermatology, let me cite the theory of positive anergy. This is an example of a hypothesis accepted on authority and faith. The theory was advanced in 1914, and over the ensuing years was passionately defended and vehemently denied. Yet, what the concept needed was neither defense nor defamation, but study and experimentation. Finally, on putting the hypothesis to a crucial test, it proved to be an immunological mirage.

Let me end with a quotation from Cicero, namely, that "Often the greatest obstacle to those who want to learn is the authority of those who teach."

DR. SUTTON continued the discussion of the paper with the following comments: If Dr. Rostenberg had spoken these words 400 years ago, he would likely have been burned at the stake, as was a great physician, Michael Servetus, in 1553 (see Garrison, 1929), while that good Christian, John Calvin, applauded. Now the fact is that almost all of us agree with Dr. Rostenberg, so we too would be burned at the stake. Times do change, apparently for the better, for I should think it a great loss if I were burned at the stake.

Re-editing this material in 1984, I wish to pursue the subject of the relationship of the Church, especially the Inquisition, to the willingness of an agile mind to inquire, to seek answers, to express opinions, and to communicate observations, such activities being the underpinnings of science as we know it, without fear of incineration.

Robert Hudson, M.D., Professor of the History of Medicine, University of Kansas Medical Center, surveyed the subject briefly for me. He quoted J. Plaidy (*The Spanish Inquisition*, New York, Citadel Press, 1967) from whom one learns that Garcia de Arias, a monk also known as "Dr. Blanco," was burned in Seville for Lutheranism September 24, 1559, but he may not have been a physician. Peter of Abano, also known as Apponensis and quoted repeatedly by Mercurialis, was more fortunate. He died—of what malady I do not know—before being adjudged guilty in about 1316. The Church, giving him their next to the best shot, burned him in effigy, the voodoo variant of ecclesiastical abracadabra that insulted his friends and relatives, vented the hatred of those who exalt love, and in no demonstrable way perturbed the still eternity of death. Encyclopaedia Britannica (12:380, 1956) mentions a medical student named Aikenhead accused of Lutheranism and hanged in Scotland in 1696.

Dr. Hudson observed that only a few victims were rather sadly used and judged that the Church got worse obloquy than in fact it earned.

This may be true, but there was significant dissuasion of thoughtful individuals who might yearn for intercommunication when it was unsafe to think and yet more unsafe to speak. One might say that curiosity was paralyzed into disuse atrophy. Day and night were created on the first day, the sun and moon on the fourth, as Genesis says, and don't ask inflammatory questions. History contains no record of which I am aware when a group of physicians blistered a churchman or two, although one might say with morbid humor that it ought in all fairness to have been done.

Let us change the subject.

It is true that one does weary of Mercurialis' endless references to the authority of the infallible Galen and the divine Plato and the Aristotelian logic whereby presumably ironclad proofs are given of what we believe to be absurdities. A good example of this is seen in Book Two, Chapter Two. I should say, nevertheless, that exposure to logic and epistemology would not harm the education of the contemporary physician. It might diminish the need, apparent in many an essay, of translating "It is logical to think" into "It is tempting to hypothesize."

Now back to the 1966 Archives of Dermatology article.

Here are several excerpts from *De Morbis Cutaneis* of Mercurialis, not all of whose words were as amusing, by our standards, as those Dr. Rostenberg selected to quote. Concerning the nature of the skin, his opening paragraph reads, "All physicians, it seems, agree that the skin has been placed about the bodies of animals as a protective covering for the flesh and members. Hippocrates in his book on bones said nature had a further purpose, that the skin is a binding for the body parts, which, being individually separate, require a common bond. It was the divine Plato who rightly likened the skin to a fisherman's net, as Galen did also."

Regarding classification, Mercurialis said, "I shall classify my material under two headings: the types of diseases peculiar to the scalp, and those common to the entire skin. The scalp, because of the brain, which is very moist and is also a major body part, is subject to particular defects, such as ophiasis, alopecia, and the like. . . . Diseases of the entire skin are of three types: those involving color, roughness or smoothness, and bulk (thickness). The diseases involving color are leuce (hypopigmentation), vitiligo, alphos (hyperpigmentation), and exanthemata. In the class of diseases of roughness and smoothness are pruritus, scabies (the scabby disease) or psora, impetigo, and lepra. In the class of diseases of bulk are papules and all skin tumors, such as acrochordons (filiform moles and warts), thymi (from Greek thymion, wart; compare thymiosis, an old synonym of frambesia), myrmecia (from Greek myrmex, ant; the disease myrmekiasis, a breaking out of warts), clavi (corns, from Latin for claws, a nail), and calluses (from Latin callosus, callous, hard)."

This classification was basically morphological, as classification continued to be until well into the twentieth century.

Concerning nomenclature and the formal presentation of medical information, he wrote, "There are five types of diseases involving the hair of the scalp: defluvium, premature calvities, canities, alopecia, and ophiasis. We have next to discuss these one by one, and in doing so we shall preserve the customary order: first we shall give the names used by physicians for the diseases; secondly, their causes and origins will be discussed; thirdly, we shall describe all the symptoms; and finally we shall disclose the best cures that can be devised."

Concerning disorders of the scalp, the following is a gem: "Caeterum de causa calvitii controversia est apud auctores"—as to the cause of baldness, there is controversy among the experts. "Hippocrates wrote that calvities is brought about by depletion of the brain, and Galen in commenting on this said that, as a man's age progresses, his brain withdraws from the cranium so that the bone, deprived of moisture, can no longer sustain hair, which, lacking nutrition, dies and falls out. . . . The causes of calvities are all those that can dry out the brain, such as insomnia, worry, late study, and immoderate coitus." Such curious, ingenuous views as to the causes and treatment of baldness persisted even into the seventeenth century (Zarca, 1973-74).

"It was Alexander of Tralles (525-605 A.D.) who suggested that calvities is actually transmitted by heredity, as gout is."

Concerning Mercurialis' "porrigo," in which I believe we would place atopic dermatitis, he wrote, "For washing either the whole body or the head, especially in the summertime, cold water is recommended, and hot water is enjoined. One must forbear anger. If anything increases the suffering in this disease it is fits of anger that make the humors boil."

Mercurialis described an interesting objective test: "Before any remedy is applied, one must ascertain whether the condition is curable. This is done by a trial of perforation. When the affected area is pricked with a needle, the kind of material that comes out is noted. If the humor that exudes is milky, this is no case for medicines because the condition is incurable; but if blood comes out, the disease will respond to medicines."

Concerning the physiology of sensation, he wrote: "In pruritus nothing comes from the skin except, as Avicenna says, some furfuraceous flakes, and not even these unless the skin is torn by the nails. Some authorities have defined pruritus as an abnormal sensation that leads to scratching, induced at a particular place from a continued dissolution due to pruritus-inciting material but without local swelling. One may say that, if it is really pruritus that this describes, then it follows that the pain due to itching and the pain of ulceration are not different. . . . From this discussion we will understand that pruritus is a symptom of the damaged action of the sense of touch . . . Socrates, as he scratched his legs confined by shackles, said that he had never experienced greater delight. I reply that even if some pleasurable sensation appears in pruritus, this is not because of the pruritus but because of the scratching. Prior to the scratching, pain is indeed manifest."

You will be interested in his prescriptions for the scabby disease and his wisdom, creditable today, regarding the use of hazardous medicines: "Medication good for scabies can be prepared as follows. Take 1 dram each of both kinds of hellebore, 1½ drams of litharge (lead oxide), 1 ounce of rose oil, ½ ounce of fresh butter, and 5 drams of bean meal. Mix carefully, and make a liniment. If a stronger preparation is desired, the following is typical. Take 1 dram each of niter (saltpeter) and brimstone. Wash three times in strong vinegar. Add ½ ounce of rose oil, 2 egg yolks, and ½ ounce of chicken fat. Mix and make a liniment . . . For getting rid of scabies, thermal baths are available, and sulfurous waters especially are likely to cure scabies promptly, after the body has been purged. It is worth considering whether quicksilver, or sublimated silver (mercury), is appropriate, for Avicenna and his followers spoke of it as marvelous. The most recent vendors of medicines (pharmacopolae, quacks) usually use this kind of medicine. On the other hand, we know that mercury is a poisonous and dangerous agent; even the Greeks do not mention it as a remedy. So I say in a scabious condition, if it is mild and recent, mercury should be entirely avoided. Great danger is involved of incorporating more of it than necessary or of using more of the ointment than is wise. Whenever a considerable hazard is involved, we must always avoid running a risk in any case that is not of itself serious. If the scabies were chronic and malignant, then we might use such medicines. They should be diluted, however, and mixed with milder agents so that we should have no great danger to fear."

It is tantalizing to attempt modern interpretations of what the ancient physicians saw, with their keen minds and alert senses. With some basic knowledge of anatomy, physiology, and microbiology, yet to be discovered, they would have looked good in the best medical company we can provide.

The bibliography follows, and then the translation of the book, with first the prefatory matter of Paulus Aicardius.

RICHARD L. SUTTON, JR.

Leawood, Kansas
July 24, 1985

BIBLIOGRAPHY

Abt-Garrison: History of Pediatrics, reprinted from Pediatrics, by various authors, edited by Abt, Isaac A., Philadelphia and London, W. B. Saunders Co., 1965.

Augusto, B. M.: Gerolamo Mercuriale, Policlinico (sezione pratica) 37:777-781, May 26, 1930.

Aulizio, Francesco: La pediatria nell' Umanesimo e nel Rinascimento con particolare riferimento a Gerolamo Mercuriale, Lattante 33:88-106, 1962.

Bellini, A.: Cenni storici sulla dermatologia in Italia; La dermatologia nell' epoca romana al rinascimento, Gior Ital Derm Sif 75:1093-1141 (June) 1934.

Belloni, L.: Streitfragen zwischen Bartolomeo Eustachi und Gerolamo Mercuriale auf dem Gebiete der medizinischen Philologie. Gesnerus 33:188-208, 1976.

Berndorfer, A.: Die Sprachstorungen im padiatrischen Wehr des Hieronimum Mercurialis vom modernen logopadischen Gesichtspunkt ausbetrachtet. Prax. Kinderpschol 8:235-8, 1959.

Bett, W. R.: Historical Note: Geronimo Mercuriale (1530-1606), Med. Press 236:307, Sept. 28, 1956.

Blundell, John W. F.: The Muscles and Their Story, from the earliest times, including the whole text of Mercurialis and the opinions of other writers ancient and modern on mental and bodily development, London, Chapman & Hall, 1864. (The text gives no indication of what is Mercurialis' and what is Blundell's. The preface indicates the difficulties of a translator.)

Boerner, F.: Noctes Guelphicae . . . de vita, morbis, meritis, et scriptis Hieronymi Mercurialis Foroliviensis commentatio, accedit duplex eiusdem eloquium alterum Jan. Nic. Erythraeo alterum Laur. Crasso auctoribus, Rostochii et Wismariae, Bergerus et Boednerus, 1755.

Boissard, J., et de Bry, T.: Icones Virorum Illustrium, Frankfurt 1597-1599, Part 3, p. 150. For text, see p. lviii.

Brambilla, G. A.: Storia d. scoperte fisico-medico-anatomico-chirurgiche fatte dagli uomini illustri Italiani . . . Milano, 1780-82, Part 2, v. 2, pp. 61-64.

Bullart: Academie des sciences et des arts, Amsterdam, 1682, v. 2, p. 112.

Busacca, A.: General Etiology and Classification of Dermatoses; Classification of Mercuriale, Folia Clinica et Biologica 12:161-171, 1940.

Busacchi, V., et al.: Numero dedicato alla memoria di Gerolamo Mercuriale, Romagna Med. 8:415-500, (Nov.) 1956.

Capparoni, Pietro: Profili Bio-Biblio-grafici di Medici e Naturalisti Celebri Itaniani Dal 15-18 centuries, Rome, Inst. Naz. medico Farmacologico "Sereno" 1928, v. 2, pp 53-56. (Includes full page copy of portrait from Collezione Gioviana degli Uffizi, in Firenze.) (See frontispiece.)

Cardini, M.: Gerolamo Mercuriale, Rivista di Storia d. scienze e naturali 21:342-345 Nov.-Dec. 1930.

Castiglione, Arturo: A History of medicine, translated from the Italian and edited by Krumbraar, E. B.: New York, Alfred A. Knopf, 2nd ed. 1947.

Cosenza, M.: Biographical and Bibliographical Dictionary of the Italian Humanists, Boston, 1962, v. 3.

Dezeimeris, O., and Raige-Delorme: Dictionnaire historique de la Médicine ancienne et moderne, Paris, v. 3, pp. 569-673.

Dondi, R. F.: La Pandemia Influenzale del 1580 nel Carteggio fra Girolamo Mercuriali e Giovanni Crattone di Kraftheim, Rivista di Storia della Medicina, 1:96-102, 1958.

Fiessinger, Ch.: La Thérapeutique des vieux maitres, Paris, Société d'Éditions Scientifiques, 1897: La Thérapeutique de Jerôme Mercuriali 1530-1606, pp. 83-89.

Garrison, Fielding H.: An Introduction to the History of Medicine, Philadelphia and London, W. B. Saunders Co., 4th ed., 1929, Mercurialis, pp. 100, 197, 207, 228; Servetus, pp. 220, 248, 754, 903.

Gnudi, M., and Webster, Jerome P.: The Life and Times of Gaspar Tagliacozzi, New York, Herbert Reichner, 1950. Engraving of Mercurialis, from Bullart (1682), faces p. 132. The book provides much biography and history of Sixteenth Century medicine, with many references to Mercurialis.

Gordon, Benjamin Lee: Medieval and Renaissance Medicine, New York, Philosophical Library, (n.d.), p. 755.

Hahn, A., Dumaitre, P., and Samion-Contet, J.: Histoire de la Médecine et du Livres Médical â la lumière des collections de la Bibliothèque de la Faculté de Médecine de Paris, Olivier Perrin, Éditeur, p. 82, p. 193.

Levinson, Abraham: Pioneers of Pediatrics, Medical Life 42:344, July, 1935.

Major, Ralph H.: A History of Medicine, Springfield, Ill., Charles C Thomas, 1954, p. 474.

Medical Greats: Jour. Amer. Med. Assn. 189:211 (Aug. 17) 1964. Brief biographic sketch with small portrait copied from Bullart (1682) which also appears in *Gnudi and Webster* (1950).

Mercuriale, Gerolamo, (1530-1606): Gior, ital. di Dermat. e Sifilog. 75:1106-

1107, 1934. (Biography with half-page reproduction of Uffizi Gallery portrait.)

Mercuriale, Gerolamo, (1530-1606): Chirurgia degli organi di movemento 2:259-274, 1918. (Biography pp. 261-266, then on De Arte Gymnastica.)

Mercuriali, Geronimo: Biographisches Lexicon der hervorragenden Arzte aller Zeiten und Völker, ed. Haberling, W., und Vierordt, H., Berlin & Wien, Urban & Schwarzenberg 2nd ed. v. 4, p. 171, 1932.

Mettler, Cecilia C.: History of Medicine, ed. by *Mettler, Fred A.* (Columbia University), Philadelphia, Blakeston Co., 1947, pp. 539, 543. (Concerned with Sixteenth Century neurology.)

Mora, George: Historical and Sociopsychiatric Appraisal of Tarantism and Its Importance in the Tradition of Psychotherapy of Mental Disorders: Bulletin History of Medicine 37:417-439, 1963. (Quotes Mercurialis' De Venenis 1584 briefly.)

Panckoucke, C.L.F. (ed.): Dictionaire des Sciences Médicales: Biographie Médicale, Paris, 1824, v. 6, pp. 255-257.

Paoletti, I.: Gerolamo Mercuriale e il suo Tempo, Cooperativa Editoriale Tipografica, Lanciano, 1963. (Sixty-two previously unpublished letters of Mercurialis, who signed his name "Hierol.^{o} Mercuriale.")

Pazzini, Adalberto: La Storia d. Facolta' Medical di Roma, Instituto di Storia d. Medicina d. Universita' di Roma, v. 2, pp. 509-510, 1961.

Perazzi, Francesco: "De Ordine Librorum Hippocratis" di Girolamo Mercuriale nelle edizioni del 1583 e del 1588, Pag. Stor. Med. 5 (2):15-24, 1961.

Perazzi, Francesco: La "Censura de Hippocratis Operibus" di Girolamo Mercurialis, Miscellanea di Studi Storica Medici 5, Instituto di Storia d. Medicine d. Univ. di Roma, 1961, 61 pp.

Ruhräh, John: Hieronymus Mercurialis 1530-1606, Amer. Jour. Dis. Child. 36: 819-821 (Oct.) 1928.

Simili, Alessandro: Storia d. Medicina, Instituto di Storia d. med. d. R. Univ. di Bologna, Gerolamo Mercuriale nell' ombra e nelle luce del suo tempo, Policlinico (sezione practica) Anno XLIX, num. 5 (Feb. 2) 1942.

Singer, Charles, and Underwood, E. A.: A Short History of Medicine, New York and Oxford, Oxford Univ. Press, 2nd ed. 1962, p. 651.

Sutton, Richard L., Jr.: The Suttons' Texts of 1916-1975 and Etiologic Classification of Diseases of the Skin, Kansas City, The Lowell Press, 1981.

Talmadge, G. Kasten: On the Influence of the Stars on Human Birth, Bull. History of Med. 13:251-267, (Mar.) 1943. (Quotes Mercurialis' De Morbis Mulieribus, 1601, re his refutation of astrologic influences on viability of eight-month fetus.)

Tomasinus, Jacob Philip: Illustrium Virorum Elogia, iconibus exornata, Padua, Donatum Pasquardum & Socium, 1630, Hieronymus Mercurialis, pp. 147-158 plus bibliography.

Zanca, A.: La calvizie nei secoli XVI e XVII, concetti etiopatogenetici e terapeutici. Acta Med. Hist. Patav. 20:105-116, 1973-74.

Zapf, Georg Wilhelm: Abbildungen berühmter und besonders um die Arzneikunde verdienter Gelehrten, nebst ihren vornehmsten Lebensumständen. Achtzehn Hefte mit 180 Porträts ... Augsburg, bey Christoph Bürglen, 1805.

Zapf dedicated his Abbildungen to Anselm Maria Fugger, Prince of the Holy Roman Empire at Babenhausen. His biographic paragraph, translated from the German script by Dr. Cora Lee Price of the University of Kansas, provided the following succinct paragraph.

Hieronymus Mercurialis was an unusually scholarly and widely recognized physician. He was born in Forli in 1530. He studied in Padua where he received the Doctor's degree. He practiced first in his native city with exceedingly gratifying success. In 1562 he entered the service of Cardinal Alexander Farnesius in Rome, and from there he went in 1569 to Padua as the first Professor of Pharmacology, and he taught there for 17 years with great recognition as both a teacher and a practitioner. He accepted a similar position at Bologna in 1585 and finally in Pisa, where he eventually received 2000 ducats annually as his salary. Since he cured Emperor Maximilian II in 1573 of a dangerous illness, the Emperor (Kaiser) not only elevated him to knighthood but also rewarded him richly. Preferring academic life, he refused the positions of personal physician offered him by many princes but returned shortly before his death to Forli and died there in 1606 of the stone.

The biographical sketch of Boissard and de Bry of 1598 is interesting in comparison. The translation was provided by Dr. Cora Lee Price.

Mercurialis, grand physician as well as accomplished in all areas of study, became the chief of the practice of medicine at the Gymnasium of Padua.

He was a native of Forli. He wrote in six books *On the Art of Gymnastics,* an activity highly prized among the ancients although largely ignored in his own day. In this work he painstakingly explained all types of ancient exercises, the manner of their performance, where they took place, the skills involved, and everything that pertains to the exercises of the human body.

He wrote also *On Diseases of the Skin and All Excrements of the Human Body,* in five books. In four books of *Various Lectures* he presented an almost endless number of passages by a great many medical writers, which he corrected where corrupt or illustrated when obscure. He edited a "Letter on Intestinal Worms" in Greek and Latin. His *Refutations* is a book in which he strenuously championed Galen in opposition to a paper by Guisandini, also a letter to Andreas Marcolinus, printed with the books of Fallopius, *On Medicinal Waters.* The second edition of his *Art of Gymnastics,* augmented by many illustrations, was printed in Paris by Jacques de Puys. He edited the four books of *Various Lectures,* and added a fifth book in which numerous passages of many writers of medicine were restored, or their obscurities elucidated. He wrote a tract *On the Plague* in which he discussed with unique learning the plague both in its general and in its specific features in Venice and Padua. Hieronymus Zanchus divided it into chapters. Mercurialis composed a book *On Adornment,* which was "useful not only to doctors and philosophers, but also to students of all branches of learning." This work was put into chapters, and to it was added the Letter of Tagliacozzi, a physician of Bologna, which contained a short but important account of restoring noses, and which was addressed to Mercurialis. He wrote a treatise on *Diseases of Children* and other books of concern to the learned.

DEDICATION TO CARDINAL SIRLETUS

AND

ADDRESS TO STUDENTS OF MEDICINE

BY

PAULUS AICARDIUS

For biographic information regarding Aicardius and Sirletus, see glossary

TO THE MOST ILLUSTRIOUS CARDINAL GULIELMUS SIRLETUS

PAULUS AICARDIUS GIVES GREETING

If one may marvel, most illustrious Cardinal, at my temerity in dedicating these works of Hieronymus Mercurialis to you whom I have never seen, one may call to mind the immensity of your virtue and excellence. No one with even a modicum of learning is unaware of the good gifts with which you abound. I should gladly recount them as in the usual dedication but for anxiety lest in my own mediocrity I might, although desiring to unfold your praises, depreciate them because of the deficiencies of my own ability.

Since the adornments of your genius have been so apparent to all that no one is astonished by their excellence, none may allege that any more perfect could be attained. I say nothing of your singular wisdom, wondrous prudence, holiness of life, and unsurpassed devotion to God, there being no need to do so; yet these are the qualities that place you in your position of dignity. Does any man exist so averse to letters and culture that he will not essay, and esteem an acquaintance with, all that is worthy, including some knowledge of the liberal arts, in which you are most learned? Upon all scholars fall your singular kindness and well-known generosity, with which you encourage them in proportion to the abundance of your riches, by which you support what you can. Hence their accomplishments appear rightly to be your own (if it is permissible to contrive great things from small ones).

Although at one time I apprehended only a fraction of your virtues, I was filled with such admiration as was, I thought, impossible to augment. Yet recently, on hearing Hieronymus Mercurialis, himself not without praise, extol with sincerity your singular talents, my devotion and regard for you increased almost beyond imagining, in witness of which I send you these works of Mercurialis, an admirer and spokesman of your great virtue, lectures that he himself considered of no great moment since they were composed during his leisure; yet they are filled with rare and recondite learning.

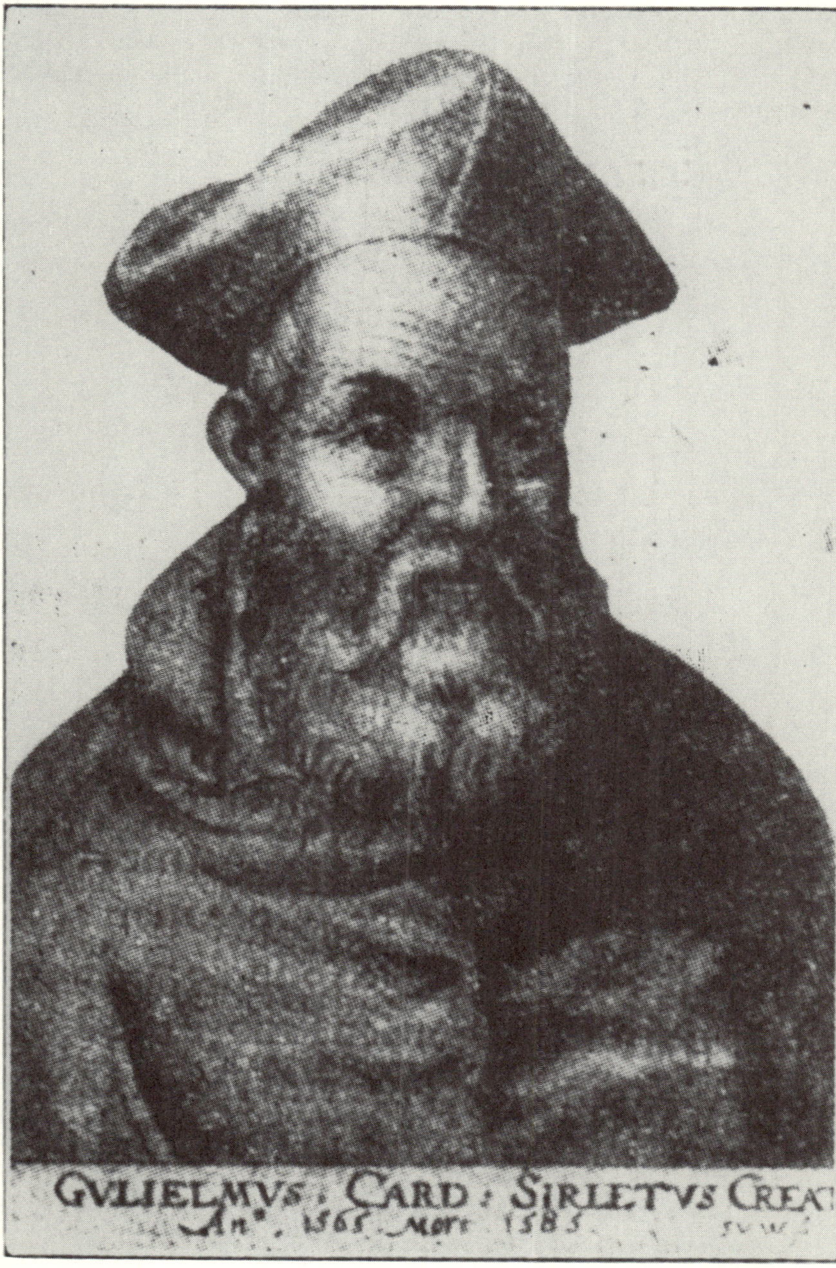
GVLIELMVS : CARD : SIRLETVS CREAT
An°. 1565. Mort 1585

I have particularly desired that these works should appear under your name, knowing that any apprehension on the part of Mercurialis would be allayed if your name were attached to this edition. So that he may know you accept these works with approval, I beg you to grant your approval if in your judgment you see fit to do so.

Padua VIII. Kal. Dec. (24 Nov.) 1571.

PAULUS AICARDIUS GIVES GREETING TO THE STUDENTS OF MEDICINE

IF I WERE not certain that few physicians in all Europe do not know who Mercurialis is, I should think it necessary to recount his virtues and proclaim the eminence of his scholarship. However, since there is no one who has not perceived his extraordinary ability, as witnessed not only by the works he himself has edited, but also by his daily lectures to throngs of listeners, I have only to relate how his lectures, casually devised on days free of classroom duties, were delivered and to explain briefly why I feel compelled to undertake this work, almost against his wishes.

After Mercurialis had been called to the celebrated Gymnasium at Rome to elucidate the sacred mysteries of Medicine, he devoted every effort to communicate all useful and necessary information. In his classroom lectures, as they are called, he so conducted himself that nothing more could be asked of him for the perfect understanding and cure of diseases, and it was apparent and generally acknowledged that such standards had not been equaled by any other professor for many years hitherto, if ever. For many of the most distinguished and ablest medical writers, such as Cornelius Celsus, Caelius Aurelianus, Theodorus Priscianus, Marcellus, Scribonius Largus, and many others, heretofore have been so generally neglected as to seem, as it were, exiled from medical schools, even though it is most disgraceful for a physician to fail to understand the many difficult passages of the outstanding authors and the discrepancies both in their own writings and with those of others. These authors seem to come alive through Mercurialis and to assume their pristine authority, for he collated what they taught along with what had been handed down by Greek and Arab physicians, and, if there were any conflicts of viewpoint, he either resolved them or, if this were not possible, judged whose opinion was preferable. In brief, he enabled anyone to become confidently intimate with all the Greek, Latin, and Arab writers. Not content with such service, he explained to his students, on days not assigned to classroom lectures, those matters which only few had comprehended or mastered.

Among his lectures are his fine essays on Diseases of the Skin and All Excrements, which have been received with such universal favor that practically everyone would wish to preserve them for himself. Many scholars, as well as learned students, have been doing this, but with a constant fault. Their notebooks are as full of inconsistencies as the writings of the ancients, for, despite their being transcribed daily, they are nevertheless perverted and distorted and lack the perfection of the original, and in fact day by day go from bad to worse.

Although aware of this, Mercurialis was quite reluctant, and gave no thought, to having the lectures printed. While many besought him to publish them, insisting that this could be done without detriment to them, and that students would benefit greatly thereby, still he could not be persuaded by the prayers or exhortations of his friends to expose his lectures to the public. He said they would be unpolished and lacking the finishing touch. When I saw that many copies were corrupted and defective, and contained nothing worthwhile, as had been transcribed by many individuals, and that these were circulated not only at Padua but among foreigners, I suggested to Mercurialis that his lectures might already have been published and that, in the condition in which they were being turned out, they might bring discredit to his name unless he himself eliminate their errors. Therefore he acquiesced, although with reservations, so that his works might be published as I should emendate them, with diligence and accuracy, and he stated that he did not wish to be completely ignorant of the undertaking. So when I had a trustworthy draft, I undertook the task of publishing it, a small enough task, but taxing to my own strength. I did this not only at the request of others, but also because my teacher, Mercurialis, considered me best equipped. After comparing many transcripts, I amended the lectures to a limited extent. I eliminated a few words, adding and detracting very little, and I did not alter the meaning of anything. This will be understood by those who have edited manuscripts. If you should come upon passages seemingly unfinished or unpolished as compared with other writings of Mercurialis, I beg you to understand that these are mere lecture notes; I need give no further explanation to those who are experienced in such matters.

Farewell, and look forward to greater things from Mercurialis, God willing.

INDEX CAPITVM SINGVLORVM LIBRORVM.

LIBRI PRIMI, DE MORBIS CVTANEIS CAPITA.

LIBRI SECVNDI.

CHAPTER INDEX OF EACH BOOK

FIRST BOOK, CHAPTERS ON DISEASES OF THE SKIN OF THE HEAD

SECOND BOOK ON DISEASES OF THE SKIN OF THE BODY

HIERONYMI MERCVRIALIS DE MORBIS CVTANEIS.

LIBER PRIMVS

CAPVT PRIMVM.

CVTEM animalium corporibus circumpoſitam eſſe, vt carnes, & membra defendat veluti tegumentum quoddam, clariſsimè conſtat apud omnes medicos. Quanquam Hippocrates in libro de oſsibus, alium finem habuiſſe Naturam in fabricanda cute dixiſſe videatur: vbi ſcribit, eam eſſe veluti quoddam membrorum ligamentum; quandoquidem cum membra ſint omnia veluti inter ſe ſeparata, opus fuit communi quodam ligamine conuinciri, quod quidem fuit cutis. Vnde fit, vt iure merito Diuinus Plato in Timæo cutim naſſulæ piſcatoriæ adſimilauerit, quod etiam adnotauit Galenus in commentarijs in Timæum. Cum itaq; ſit hic ſolus cutis vſus, cumque nullam aliam actionem vtilem habeat, ſed ſolum excrementorum ſit receptaculum, vt docuit Galenus lib. de cauſsis morborum cap. VI. Ea propter paucis morbis obnoxia eſt: de quibus omnibus propoſitum eſt nobis verba facere. Totam autem tractationem hanc in duo capita partiar, in ea morborum genera, quæ capiti particularia ſunt, & in ea, quæ vniuerſæ cuti ſunt communia. Capitis enim cutis ob cerebrum, quod & humidisſimum, & maximum membrum eſt, peculiaribus quibuſdam vitijs obnoxia fuit, qualia ſunt ophiaſis, alopecia, & ſimilia. Hi uerò morbi, quos cutis eſſe dicimus, ſunt vitia vel capillorum, vel totius cutis capitis. Vitia capillorum ſunt ophiaſis, defluuium, alopecia, caluitium, & canities: cutis autem, vlcera manantia, & ſicca, quemadmodum docebimus ſuo loco. Neque mirum ſit, quòd dixerim, vitia capillorum eſſe morbos cutis capitis; quandoquidem, vt habemus à Galeno xiiij. Methodi cap. xviij. capilli capitis nequaquam corporis partes ſunt, ſed potius particulæ quædam, & ſunt veluti quædam adnata cuti, facta à Natura ob duos fines, vt docet idem Galenus lib. xj. de vſu partium cap. xiiij. vnus vſus eſt, vt & gene-

BOOK ONE, CHAPTER ONE

HIERONYMUS MERCURIALIS ON DISEASES OF THE SKIN

THE SKIN, all physicians apparently agree, has been placed about the bodies of animals as a protective covering for the flesh and members. Hippocrates in his book on bones seems to have said that nature had a further purpose in providing skin. He wrote that it is a binding for the body parts, which, being individually separate, require a common bond, and this is the skin. Thus the divine Plato rightly likened the skin to a fisherman's net, as Galen did also. Since this is the only function of the skin, which has no other use save as a receptacle for waste materials, as Galen taught, it is subject to a variety of diseases, all of which I intend to discuss.

I shall classify them under two headings: the types of diseases peculiar to the scalp, and those affecting the entire skin.

The scalp, because of the brain, is very moist, and it is also a major body part, subject to particular defects, such as ophiasis, alopecia, and the like. Diseases we consider to be of the skin are affections either of the hair or of the whole scalp. Hair affections are ophiasis, defluvium, alopecia, calvities, and canities. In the proper place we shall discuss the moist and the dry ulcers of the skin of the scalp.

That hair affections are "diseases" of the skin of the head, as I stated, should not seem strange, for we have it from Galen that the hair of the scalp is by no means a primary structure but rather an attachment to, or an appendage of, the skin, made by nature for two purposes, as Galen taught: by its growth and nourishment it purifies the head of excrement and provides for dignity of appearance and adornment.

Since hair exists for these two purposes, I believe I am correct in stating that abnormalities of the hair are diseases of the skin, for hair does not suffer unless the skin itself or the humors contained in it are adversely affected. One may wonder how this can be true when Aristotle asked why, where there is vitiligo, the hair is white, but not vice versa, as if necessarily the hair might be abnormal apart from abnormality of the skin. The explanation is that the hair is influenced by a diseased skin, but that the converse is not true. I suggest that the skin may be thought of as skin alone or the whole of the skin along with its appendages and the humors contained in it. If the first alternative were accepted, then hair might be affected by what does not affect the skin, as remarked by Aristotle; but if the latter is assumed, then it must be said that the hair cannot be abnormal unless the skin is also. Aristotle stated that the skin of the head is extremely thick and full of humors.

It seems to me that diseases of the entire skin are of three types: those of color, of roughness or smoothness, and of bulk. The diseases involving color are leuce, vitiligo, alphos, and exanthemata. In the class of diseases of roughness and smoothness are pruritus, scabies, or psora, impetigo, and lepra. In the class of diseases of bulk are papules and all skin tumors, such as acrochordons (filiform moles), thymi (Gr thymion, wart: thymiosis, an old synonym of frambesia), myrmecia (Gr myrmex, ant; the disease myrmekiasis, a breaking out of "warts"), clavi (L clavus, a nail; corns), and calluses (L callosus, callous, hard).

All of these kinds of skin diseases we shall discuss, given sufficient time; but regarding them, uncertainties arise. The first is that, Hippocrates wrote, lepra, scabies, pruritus, and alopecia are "disfigurements" (turpitudines) rather than "diseases." If this is true, it is incorrect, I suppose, to class them as diseases. Furthermore, according to Galen, the skin has no independent actions and so is not subject to diseases, which are derangements of actions. The second question concerns my class of diseases involving skin color, for Galen seems not to have recognized such; nor perhaps should this be done, for color, however it may be changed, will never harm actions.

As to the first question, Hippocrates did not deny that lepra (of the Greeks, psoriasis) and scabies are diseases, but he stated, too, that they are essentially disfigurements. In lepra and scabies, if the disorders of actions they cause are compared with the disfigurements they cause, the latter are undoubtedly more conspicuous.

It is reasonable to say that the body parts have two functions, the one common and useful to all parts, the other individual. As Galen stated, the skin does not have common functions; its functions are neither necessary nor useful to any body part. It does have its individual actions. We know that it receives nourishment from the veins, nourishment which the skin must of necessity attract, assimilate, unite, and distribute. Since these functions not rarely become abnormal in the skin, it is not unreasonable to believe that their abnormalities are diseases.

Many believe that such diseases of the skin should be termed diseases of appearance or of comeliness (pulchritude). I consider this wholly hypothetical because, if a disease of pulchritude were assumed to exist, Galen would necessarily have been deceptive, for he nowhere mentioned such a thing. If it did exist, comeliness would be health, and, since it is found even in bodies that are not living, we should feel obligated to say that health is found in dead bodies, which is false, for Aristotle stated that health and disease occur only in the living.

Aware that these uncertainties might arise, we must clarify them here before trying to solve the second difficulty. Galen wrote that it is the duty of physicians to be informed about comeliness and its opposite, but medicine is versed primarily in disease and health; hence those features are, respectively, health and disease. Also, Plato wrote that turpitude is simply the disharmony of related things. Disease is a disharmony of this type. Thus turpitude is disease, and consequently pulchritude is health.

If Galen in any of his writings made a distinction, he did state that comeliness is the fruit of health and is concurrent with health and strength in a sound body. In my view, the physician is concerned with form and deformity, not primarily or solely, but consequentially. He is primarily concerned with health and illness, and, as pulchritude is the fruit of health, as Galen said, so disfigurement is the fruit of illness. It is from this point of view that Galen wrote that medical men and the medical arts are concerned with form and deformity.

I must say of Plato's views, it is not true that because deformity is disharmony, therefore it is also disease, for Galen himself clearly distinguished form from health when he spoke of the symmetry of the limbs as "this consonance of humors and the limbs."

As for the second difficulty concerned with whether abnormality of color constitutes disease, I know that some authorities presently believe that abnormality of color merely indicates disease, yet I am persuaded in my view by the fact that an abnormal color of the membrane of the eye may damage vision. This is not the place to dispute the matter.

I describe diseases involving the color of the skin for two reasons: first, because the symptoms are commonly given disease names, and, secondly, a disease of the skin may be manifested by color changes only. When the nutritive capability of the skin is impaired, the color is changed immediately (without intervening cause, not mediately), as occurs in vitiligo. As soon as the color does change, the skin is recognized as suffering disease. As Aristotle wrote, the skin whitened by disease differs from skin naturally white, just as hairs whitened by disease differ from those that whiten naturally.

BOOK ONE, CHAPTER TWO

ON DISEASES OF THE SKIN OF THE HEAD ACCORDING TO CLASSES

LET US BEGIN by discussing disorders of the scalp rather than of the skin in general, for, as Galen wrote, however one may describe diseases of the body, one must begin with the head as its most august part. The hairs of the head come from burned and sooty waste, which nature expels through the skin and which, as it coheres and extends in length, assumes the form of hair not only because of its materia but also because of the strait passageway through which it is discharged. Thus all abnormalities of the hair result from abnormalities of its substance (materia) or of the pores through which it is naturally expelled.

Abnormalities of substance come about because it is scarce, wanting, or defective. Scarcity occurs if the hair is not fed and if its materia is not supplied. Hair is maintained by a continuous influx of the humors, an insufficiency of which would result in a deficiency of the hair.

Hair may be diminished as an incident of illness, for there are many diseases, such as phthisis and cachexia, in which the excrements that maintain the hair are not formed, so that the hair, deprived of the humors, easily dies. We see this in plants, too, when inadequately nourished, they dry up and die. An insufficiency of excrements occurs when moisture is consumed, as in calvities, when body moisture is used up.

Excrements cannot be supplied when for some reason the brain shrinks. As long as the brain fills the cranium, it moistens the whole of the scalp and maintains its nutrition. If the brain withdraws from the cranium, the skin will lack an abundance of moisture and will be unable to supply the hair with the necessary nutrient. Aristotle said that this may come about through coitus. If indeed the brain declines in people who overindulge and recedes from the cranium, a balding process will quickly follow. Hippocrates indicated this when he mentioned "consumption of the brain and consequent baldness."

Disorders of the hair result from destruction of excrements, when excrementary moisture is so used up that nothing is left for maintenance of the hair. Similarly we see plants growing in sandy soil unable long to survive because they have no nutrient that they can use.

Abnormalities of the hair result from abnormal kinds of excrements, either because these have themselves been corrupted without complication, or because they have been corrupted by abnormal and malignant (injurious) conditions. If they have been corrupted without complication, canities ensues. I refer to the canities resulting from disease as was recognized by Aristotle and confirmed by Avicenna, who called it the "canities of youth."

Disorders involving corrupted excrement differ from deformed and injurious abnormalities of it in two ways. Either all the capilli are impaired—the word "alopecia" is said to be derived from "fox" (Gr alopex; alopos, like a fox), animals generally susceptible to this kind of disease—or else not all the hair, but some of it, falls out, a condition called ophiasis, or "tyria," derived from the word (Gr phtheir, louse) for creeping, crawling things, as we shall elaborate upon in the proper place. These conditions are both given the same name, "areae," by Cornelius Celsus. They may result not only from the Gallic disease (syphilis) but also from ulcers and other causes which we shall duly elucidate.

Disorders involving the hair due to abnormalities of the pores result from either their excessive density or excessive laxity. The pores of the skin become narrow either because of exsiccation, so that they are closed up and unable to provide a passageway for the sooty excrement and hence the hair falls out, or because the skin becomes indurated, as in the scars of wounds or ulcers that have healed, especially in ulcerative tinea. In such cases the skin becomes indurated to such an extent that moisture is unavailable to preserve the hair. Disorders occur also because of looseness (latitudo). Just as trees cannot persevere and thrive in thin earth, so also hairs cannot endure in thin and lax skin. Galen seems to have called this particular condition "defluvium."

So we conclude that there are five types of diseases involving the hair of the scalp: defluvium, premature calvities, canities, alopecia, and ophiasis. We have next to discuss these one by one, and in doing so we shall preserve the customary order: first, we shall give the names used by physicians for the diseases. Secondly, their causes and origins will be discussed. Thirdly, we shall describe all the symptoms, and finally we shall disclose the best therapy that can be devised.

BOOK ONE, CHAPTER THREE

ON DEFLUVIUM OF THE HAIR

BEFORE beginning the discussion of defluvium, it is helpful to note that not all writers have discussed hair diseases one by one. Paulus described only calvities, alopecia, and ophiasis. Oribasius and Aetius described alopecia, canities, calvities, and ophiasis. Rhazes mentioned ophiasis, canities, and alopecia in its advanced stage only. Galen and Avicenna apparently described all the diseases of the hair that I intend to. One must recognize that "defluvium" is a name commonly used for diverse conditions. Sometimes it signifies the particular condition I shall consider here.

Defluvium actually means nothing more than the falling out of hair due, not to abnormality of the humors as in alopecia, but to other causes, which we shall consider later. While it may occur under other circumstances, Galen believed that it occurs most frequently after prolonged illness. More or less of the hair may fall. Obviously only rarely is the scalp entirely depilated.

The causes, according to Galen, are two: thinness (raritas) of the scalp pores, and dearth of the materia that generates and nourishes the hair. As plants cannot survive in thin earth, so the hair is affected when the scalp is thinned. Like plants in earth that is arid and lacks humor, the hair, too, cannot be nourished when the skin is not.

Theodorus Priscianus and Actuarius advocated the view that defluvium results from an excess of the humors, for Plato said that plants often wither (arescunt) when they are overnourished, such as may occur in marshes and swamps. So also hairs, sometimes overnourished, are as it were suffocated and die. Alexander of Tralles attributed defluvium to two other causes, thickness (condensation, density) of the skin, and excretion of abnormal humors.

It may be asked how defluvium can result from thickness when Galen said it results rather from rarefaction. The argument is not absurd, since it is possible for the skin, as a result of medication or other causes, to become so puckered and condensed that nutrition of the hair cannot be maintained, and after awhile the hair, deprived of nutrient, falls out. It is inconsistent to insist that hair falls out only because of abnormality of the humors, as it does in alopecia, or because of its eliminating abnormal humors, as Alexander said, for in alopecia the hair roots are destroyed by an abnormality of the fluid. As to the cause suggested by Alexander, the pores are opened by the outflow and elimination of the abnormal humors, and so the hair falls out. Marcellus preferred to believe that the hair falls out because of a malfunction.

Quintus Serenus, the physician, ascribed the falling of hair to two other causes, the drinking of poisons and the touch of the salamander, in eloquent verse, the truth of which one cannot doubt:

> "The hair falls out, expelled by lurking disease, if seldom washed; and by power of poison quaffed or touch of potent salamander, impervious to flame, will the crowning glory be defiled."

All these causes for defluvium have been given by medical authorities.

Defluvium that originates from defective nutrition is recognized principally by looking into the dietary habits, such as the starvation endured by a sick patient. It is also recognized as resulting from prolonged fatigue or excessive coitus, which result in defluvium because the hair is deprived of nutrient. Such debilitating conditions may indicate the cause in defluvium, and, while Galen said it rarely occurs in the absence of disease, yet this can occur. If hair falls out from rarefaction alone, it is recognized usually by the patient's temperature since the scalp will be hot, loose, and open, and the patient sweats a great deal, particularly about the head. If caused by the density of the skin, the same changes are seen: the hair will be frail, tightened as it were, and compacted. The skin is similarly affected in patients who are excessively exposed to cold or who have used strong astringents.

As to prognosis, Hippocrates wrote that, if the hair falls because of wasting due to diarrhea, death will surely ensue. Galen, in his comment on this passage, concurred because the loss of hair in wasting sickness shows that nature has been influenced profoundly by the inadequacy of nutrition.

When hair falls because of nutritional deficiency, it is interesting to speculate on the statement of Aristotle that, often in wasting illnesses and even in dead bodies, the hair sometimes grows. Both Aristotle and Averroes appear to have accepted the explanation that, in both sick and emaciated patients, much excrement is produced, since the body parts are fed; hence the materia for the growth and increment of the hair is amply supplied.

As to how the hair may increase in the dead, where rather it ought to fall out, Averroes and John the Grammarian remained silent. I suspect they did not believe what Aristotle said. Some who have attempted to explain it have argued that in the dead a great corruption occurs so that quantities of excrement are brought forth, wherefore the hair may readily grow and increase. This interpretation seems unfounded and ridiculous to me because, not merely is an abundance of excrement necessary to promote the growth of hair, but also an active agency is needed for expelling it, and this is absent in the dead. Thus we cannot accept this explanation.

Plotinus wrote that the hair and fingernails of the dead grow because, even if anima withdraws, nevertheless a vestige of it remains for some time as a kind of life indeed capable of growing hair, just as, after a fire has burned out, we note that heat remains at the site for some time. This view does not seem creditable to me because, as the body undergoes decay, this decay pervades the entirety of the prima materia, so that no life and no faculty of the soul remain. As when the sun sets, its rays and all its light recede, so also when anima leaves the body, all its faculties depart; and so this view of Plotinus seems untrue. I would point out that Alexander of Tralles wrote that in death, when the flesh is decaying, the hairs become exposed to their roots so that they seem to be longer but not because they are growing or increasing in any way. This is evidently Aristotle's meaning when he said that the hair does seem to lengthen after death but is not generated. As long as a creature is living, the hairs are not elongating but rather are continually being generated.

Let us now consider the treatment of defluvium, the therapeutic purposes of which, Galen said, differ from those in curing alopecia. In alopecia, the humors must be purged and the skin cleansed. In defluvium, however, nothing should be done but to increase the firmness of the skin moderately and to supply food for generating hair. First, then, a dietary regimen should be established so efficacious that, as Galen taught, the disease may be cured by diet alone. So if defluvium arises from rarefaction of the skin, astringent foods should be given that are optimally nourishing and readily digested. Pure astringent wine is an extremely useful food of this type, as are also citron, pomegranate, meats that nourish particularly well, egg yolk, and other foods of the kinds that condense the skin. Some recommend kid's feet or the feet of the young bull calf. If defluvium comes on because of condensation of the skin, or dryness, which is almost the same, Alexander of Tralles recommended the use of the bath, which I also endorse. Advantageous also are moistening herbs, fruits, and all the things capable of rarefying the skin moderately.

It is to be noted that in any kind of hair loss one must never use too many rarefying agents, which, even if they may promote that generation of hair which is lacking, are nevertheless injurious to the preservation of hair that has not as yet fallen out.

Medicines to be taken internally are unnecessary in this illness and have not been proposed by Galen or any other authority, but external agents are necessary. These should have the property of strengthening the skin and of conveying nutrient to it, especially when defluvium comes from rarefaction of the skin. A medicament of this kind is labdanum, highly recommended by Galen. One must not suppose that this was Galen's discovery, for Hippocrates wrote that labdanum is especially useful in defluvium, along with rose oil or anethine oil. He also praised cimolian earth, along with omphacine oil and rose oil, wine, and acacia. Ointments and lotions for the scalp may be prepared from astringent and strengthening agents of this type, such as juniper and lentiscus.

In the correct use of these, Galen taught that three essentials must always be observed. One is that, if time permits, all the hair should be removed, for two reasons: if it is not, the medicament cannot be used properly; and, as Cornelius Celsus wrote, shaving the head is beneficial. Two methods are available for removing hair, according to Galen: shaving with a razor and plucking with forceps, which latter he seems to have preferred. The second essential is that medicament should not be applied to hair that is falling unless the head has first been massaged, because this strengthens the scalp and more nutrient is carried to it. The third essential is that, if the head is shaved, the medications should be rather thick, whereas if the scalp is plucked, they should be more liquid.

We give the composition of two lotions, one for thickened skin, the other for rarefied. The following is for the latter. Take 5 pounds of oak ash lye, 2 handfuls of lentiscus, 1½ handfuls of rose leaves, 1 handful of myrtle berries, and 2 drams each of labdanum and acadia mixed together. These are boiled until a third is consumed, then allowed to stand. Then the head is treated with this wash. The lotion for thickened skin is as follows. Take 6 pounds of lye of grape vine ash, 2 handfuls each of leaves of camomile and melilot, 1½ handfuls of lentiscus, 1 handful of rose leaves, and 3 drams each labdanum and malabathrum tied in a small bundle. Boil these until a third is consumed. Strain carefully and apply the wash to the head. Note that although the skin is thickened, nevertheless I use not only relaxing and aperient agents but also moderately astringent ones. After the scalp wash has been used, then an ointment is applied.

I will describe the three ointments and medicaments I use with great success. The first is made from distilled oil of labdanum. I take 2 parts of labdanum and 1 part of myrtle berries, and prepare the oil with an alembic (by distillation). Along with the lotion, I use this oil with great success on rarefied skin. I have another kind of oil that I make in a particular way. Take 2 drams of green nut shell juice, 1½ ounces each of oil of labdanum and oil of myrtle, 1 dram each of myrtle powder and mastic powder, and an equal amount of beeswax. Mix over a fire, and make an ointment.

Many other types of ointments can be found in the writings of Galen and other authors. If the skin is puckered (adstricta), I usually use oil of labdanum for this, and incorporate a bit of cinnamon and malabathrum. For example, take 2 ounces of oil of extracted labdanum, 1 dram of cinnamon, and 1½ drams of malabathrum or a substitute. Add a bit of beeswax, mix, and make a liniment.

For winter and cold weather Galen, we see, recommended three ointments, nardicum, spicatum, and foliatum. The nardine ointment, as we have it according to Theophrastus and Dioscorides, consisted of the juice of the roots of the nard itself. Spicatum was from spikenard. Some have thought that foliatum consisted of nard leaves, hence so called (L folium, leaf), but this is untrue, for we know from Dioscorides that the oil was called "foliatum." Besides nard, these authorities included malabathrum, by some called "folium"; so according to them the oil of malabathrum and foliatum were the same.

As for the compositions of the ointments, I regularly use the ingredients found among our ointment makers, oil of roses, oil of spike, and sometimes oil of caryophyllus (cloves), although quite rarely, because it is too hot and, if not diluted, makes the scalp too hot and too loose. We might use the following liniment in the winter and cold weather. Take ½ or 1 ounce each of spike oil and oil of roses, 1½ drams each of labdanum and finely powdered malabathrum, and beeswax sufficient to make a liniment.

One may wonder why I put labdanum in all the liniments. As may be seen in Galen, it has a moderate power of condensing and of attracting nourishment to the hair. Labdanum is the outstanding remedy for falling hair.

Marcellus and Priscianus mentioned many other medicines that I omit.

BOOK ONE, CHAPTER FOUR

ON ALOPECIA AND OPHIASIS

THERE ARE four kinds of diseases of the capilli (hairs of the scalp), as I have said, defluvium, alopecia, ophiasis, and calvities. We have discussed defluvium, so we turn next to alopecia and ophiasis, both in one chapter. While these two conditions involve the same materia, nevertheless they differ, as Galen taught, with respect to their configuration. In alopecia the head is almost completely without hair; in ophiasis, only certain areas, of the shape of snake tracks, hence the name, "ophiasis" (Gr ophis, snake). Cornelius Celsus spoke of both conditions as "areae." Galen stated that Hippocrates called them "phalakrosis" and "madarosis" (Gr adj applicable to flesh as flaccid or loose, to scalp, bald), i.e., calvities. These conditions represent hair loss from erosion of the roots by the decay of the humors.

One may ask why Aristotle wrote that alopecias are corruptions and alterations of the superfices of the skin. I should say Aristotle's interpretation is correct, for in alopecia some kind of abnormality must pervade the whole skin while affecting it only superficially. Alopecia and ophiasis, according to Celsus, have several features in common. The hair is weakened at the surface of the scalp and, when sufficiently weakened, falls out; if the site is bruised, blood of foul odor and a liquid exude; and the disease progresses rapidly in some cases, slowly in others.

One must give thought to what the causes are and why a certain tortuosity appears in ophiasis. Avenzoar, a writer of the greatest authority, undertook an explanation. He thought the tortuosity in ophiasis is simply because the materia is rather thick. Comparably, when pure water is tossed onto the pavement, it flows in a straight line, but if mud is added and the mixture is splashed on the ground, it will splash in curves and loops. He must be right, for as long as the corrupted phlegm is thin, it destroys the hair in straight lines, but if a thick materia is intermixed, it corrupts the humors deviously.

Blood, phlegm, yellow bile, and black bile can all give rise to these diseases, as Galen wrote; hence there are as many varieties of them as there are of materia. The variations are severally recognized by their particular symptoms, especially by their color, for, as Hippocrates taught, colors indicate dominant humors. Galen said that as long as the body is healthy the colors of the hair are natural, but when the body is defective, the hair develops colors in accordance with the qualities of the dominant humors. Thus we recognize that alopecia and ophiasis are of sanguine origin if the color of the skin is reddish, and they come from phlegm if the color is white, from melancholy if the color is livid, and from bile if the color is pallid or grayish-white.

We must note another point, made by Actuarius, on how hairs grow back. If the regenerated hairs are of various colors, the materiae that bring this about must be various.

There is a contradiction between the Greek writers and Cornelius Celsus, for, as we have said, Galen and his followers recognized no difference between ophiasis and alopecia other than the configuration. But Celsus gave many other distinctions: alopecia areata spreads in a particular configuration, may involve the beard, may affect patients of any age, and seldom heals without medical attention; but ophiasis begins in the back of the head, never exceeds a width of two fingers, extends to both ears simultaneously, spreads to the front of the head and returns back again, and is often cured without medical effort, particularly when it occurs in children. I, too, therefore think it clear that many differences exist between the two diseases. Avenzoar added that alopecia results from larger amounts of, and more thickly compacted, phlegmatic materia; and this in ophiasis is lesser in amount and more fluid. Quintus Serenus, an authority not to be dismissed lightly, described ophiasis eloquently in these words:

> "Sometimes the patches vary, and from time to time new lesions develop in the form of small ringlets."

To eliminate this contradiction, I think it must be said that Cornelius Celsus, in view of the aforementioned distinctions, was indeed more painstaking than the Greek writers. Galen was content to ascribe the same material cause to both diseases, and from it the indications for treatment might be deduced.

As to prognosis, Hippocrates wrote that in the scalp large vessels (varices) develop, through the influence of which the hairs are regenerated, an opinion in which Aristotle concurred. Here Galen said that the grand old man, Hippocrates, mistook the true meaning of "calvities" by including within it alopecia and ophiasis, when he said that in the brain is much phlegm, which is corrupted when agitated by coitus so that it leaves the hair roots, thereby causing calvities. Galen would teach that in ophiasis and alopecia, if enlarged vessels are present, the hair will be regenerated.

Among more recent writers, some who disagree with Galen are of the opinion Hippocrates in this instance did not misconstrue the true meaning of calvities. They say calvities is actually of two kinds, the one being that due to old age, which can never be cured, the other being independent of old age and capable of undergoing spontaneous natural cure. They say there are some illnesses that respond to medical art and are cured by nature, such as dislocated joints, and others cured by nature but not by art, such as, for example, calvities. They say, furthermore, an indication that calvities can be cured is the presence of varices, which were considered to be "contraries" of calvities by Hippocrates. If contraries were cured by contraries, it would be easy to understand how calvities might undergo spontaneous cure. But this seems fatuous to me because in the works of no medical authority is calvities to be found except with the meaning of a defluvium in which hair falls out because of a substantial deficiency of moisture. Since in true calvities this moisture cannot be restored naturally, the disease is necessarily incurable; therefore Hippocrates could not have been discussing this type of calvities.

Ophiasis, according to Avenzoar, is easier to cure than alopecia, but Serapion held the contrary opinion. I think alopecia is far more difficult to cure than ophiasis because the materia of alopecia is more copious and thicker. Because of these two reasons alopecia is more recalcitrant and more resistant. Not without justification Cornelius Celsus said that ophiasis can be cured readily, alopecia almost never. In this connection, Pliny the physician, under whose name we have four books on medicine, wrote that alopecia is a markedly degrading and unclean disease and that slaves with alopecia have always sold at a lower price.

We now reach consideration of the treatments that Galen said are most important. First, the body must be cleansed of abnormal and corrupt humors. Secondly, medicines are to be administered that are capable of regenerating the already corrupted hair. If the body is not previously purified and we attempt to regenerate hair, we should clearly be wasting our efforts. As Theodorus Priscianus, the physician, said, the hair that is regenerated would be like fruit nourished by defective earth juices.

Because defective juices accumulate in the body either from defective nutrition or from some other disorder of the whole body, of the liver, or of the scalp, therefore before anything else is undertaken a dietary regimen must be established. The foods to be eaten are those that best give rise to good juices and are easily digested, such as wine that is light, watery, and neither rich nor thick. Venery must be avoided and also exertions of the body, prior to purgation, because, as we are taught both by Theophrastus and by Galen in many passages, if impure bodies are stimulated, they become readily subject to sores. The bowels should be kept loose, and the patient's way of life should be regulated so as to promote good health (a favorable disposition). People handicapped by a poor condition (adfectionis) will always live a defective life. In patients who have lost hair from the Gallic disease, it frequently appears that, to the extent they live the more happily, to that extent they are cured the more quickly.

After establishing the diet, we must consider the purgation of the body. The appropriate method will be indicated by the nature of the dominant humor. If it is blood that causes the disease, the initial treatment should be the letting of blood, not omitting, however, the loosening of the bowels. Blood should be withdrawn in such an amount as will not impair strength. When blood is superabundant, the interior elbow vein should be incised. If the left side seems more affected, blood should be drawn from the left side; if the right, then from the right.

After blood has been let, we proceed with purgation, to be accomplished with the best decoctions and appropriate syrups. Take 1 handful each of hop leaves, bugloss, borage, and melissa, and make a decoction. To 5 ounces of this, add 1 ounce each of syrup of hops and syrup of borage juice. Mix. This is the formula for treating the sanguineous cases.

The medicines for purging distorted humors if any elements of blood are intermixed ought to be smooth and gentle. They should never be overdone (transeatur). Suitable are manna, syrup of violet solution, or syrup of rose solution.

If the materia is phlegmatic, bloodletting should be entirely omitted.

Next comes medication for the phlegm, for which the following is suitable. Take 1 handful each of leaves of betony, stechados, origanum, and marjoram. Make a decoction in the usual manner. To 5 ounces of the mixture add 1 ounce each of simple oxymel, syrup of betony, and syrup of stechados. Mix. When this has been prepared appropriately, the phlegm will be purged.

In these cases Galen praised highly the hiera of colocynth in pill form. It is best to use this with either hiera of Pacchius or hiera of Archigenes.

One must note that medicines for diseases of the scalp should always be given in pill form, for, if it is necessary to purge the head, this form of medication is most appropriate for drawing corrupt humors from the head.

If the materia is bilious, the following potion may be prepared. Take 1 handful each of leaves of endive, plantain, lactuca, and chickory. Make a decoction. To 5 ounces of this mixture add 1 ounce each of syrup of endive and syrup of portulaca or of lactuca, and mix.

For purging bile, pills of rhubarb are suitable, or any pill containing scammony, which purges bile effectively. Aloes may be added. Such medicine will be suitable. As Galen and Mesue wrote, it purges bile wonderfully well.

If the materia is melancholic, the following medicine should be prepared. Take 1 handful each of leaves of fumitory, scolopendrium, borage, and sorrel. Make a decoction. To 5 ounces of this mixture, add 1 ounce each of syrup of fruit juice and syrup of fumitory juice. Mix. For purging melancholia, pills of lapis lazuli are suitable, pills of fumitory, or of cochiae with hellebore.

These will purge every kind of humor that causes alopecia or ophiasis.

After purging the humors, and because most of the effective medication in these diseases lies in topical applications, we now come to the discussion of those agents which, as Galen taught, must have three properties. First and foremost, they must have the power to break up, evacuate, and dissipate heavy humors (must be discutient, evacuant, and dissipative). This cannot readily be done unless outstanding dispersive power is present. However, such medicines are usually hot, and, since they drive out healthy elements, they are apt to compact and destroy the hair. One must be chary of using hot remedies. The second necessary property is that of penetrating to the depths of the skin. Thirdly and finally, they must be able to draw forth from the body the best and most suitable blood supply (ambitu) for the regeneration and nutrition of the hair.

Galen and other physicians have taught that these three properties are to be found in thapsia, a medicine therefore to be used frequently. Since thapsia is hotter, however, than is suitable, Galen warned that it must be diluted with either a simple savin oil or pure water.

Why in this condition does one not adhere to the therapeutic procedure usual for other diseases characterized by the flux of materia, in which first repellent and then dispersive agents are used? Galen explained that, at the onset of alopecia or ophiasis, the physician ought to use repellents but is not consulted then; rather, he is consulted after the condition has developed, so it is unnecessary to discuss repellent medication. Then, too, the cause of alopecia is distinct from alopecia itself. So we will discuss alopecia and ophiasis themselves rather than their incipient stages.

Topical medicines should be discutient, penetrant, and capable of calling forth the best blood. But as we have said, because the materiae are diverse that give rise to these diseases, various medicinals appropriate for each must be selected forthwith.

If the case is phlegmatic, the following liniment is best. Take 4 drams each of euphorbium and wild rue and 1½ drams each of sulfur and white hellebore. Mix with an aged nut oil to make a liniment. The nut oil is included because Avenzoar, the great experimentalist, found that it works wonders in these conditions.

If the materia is bilious, a different liniment is more suitable. Take ½ ounce each of alconium, burned bitter almonds, roots of the red canna, and mouse dung (stercoris murium). Mix with vinegar and chicken fat to make an ointment.

If the materia is melancholic, the following should be used. Take 1 dram of thapsia (washed with water), 2 drams of burned abrotanum, 3 drams each of burned hazel bark and fly heads (heads of cantharides; see last paragraph of this chapter), 2 drams of cantharides, and rose oil sufficient to make a liniment. This is rather strong because the melancholic humor is more stubborn than the others.

Finally, if the materia is sanguineous, the following medicine is suitable. Take 2 drams of labdanum, 1 ounce of egg yolk oil, and 2 drams each of paper ash and ash of salted fly heads. Make an ointment with old olive oil.

As to the use of these medicines, one must always remember four things. First, as taught by Alexander of Tralles, in cases of briefer duration the milder medicines should be used; in chronic cases, the more potent ones. Secondly, before the lesions are anointed, the diseased hairs must be plucked out carefully. As farmers remove rotten and useless roots before they sow seed, so before we seek regeneration of the hair we should remove the corrupt and useless hairs; otherwise hair will not sprout, or that which does, will be corrupt.

There are two ways to remove diseased hairs. The first, requiring clear, bright light, is to remove them one by one with tweezers. Considerable diligence is needed to do this, for the operation requires both time and skill. The other, used since ancient times, is to apply pitch to the diseased area. Adhering to the hairs, this takes the diseased ones with it when it is pulled off. These methods cannot be performed without some pain and trauma.

The third point is that, after the corrupt hairs have been epilated and before applying liniment, the area must be rubbed until the skin is red. Friction can be applied in various ways. A rough piece of cloth may be used, or pumice, saltpeter, fig leaves, or radish or onion root. Whatever is handy is all right and is to be applied vigorously to the depilated area until it is made red. After that, the liniment is applied.

The fourth point concerns the use of thapsia and cantharides. Galen says that discrimination is needed in the selection of thapsia. When new it is strong, after a year weaker, and after three years still weaker. That which is one year old should be diluted; that which is two years old, diluted less; and by the time it is three years old, it needs little or no correction. In using thapsia, one must keep these facts in mind.

As to the use of cantharides, the great Hippocrates advised that the head, wings, and feet should be cut off. Dioscorides and Pliny were of the opinion that these external parts of the fly are, as it were, a protection for their bodies, a point noted by Galen, who stated he sometimes used cantharides made of the whole insect, not only as a topical medication but also internally. In preparing it, I prefer to use the whole insect. Since it is to be applied externally, it is not dangerous, and it works better as a discutient and enables other medication to penetrate into the depths of the skin.

BOOK ONE, CHAPTER FIVE

ON CALVITIES

CALVITIES, called by the Greeks "phalacrosis" or "madarosis," is simply the hair loss that occurs in old men. I say "old" because defluvium, which we discussed in Chapter Three, is also hair loss from the scalp but differs a good deal from the calvities that is the subject before us.

Defluvium occurs at any age and in both sexes, involves the whole of the head, and results from many causes. True calvities occurs only at a particular time of life, and its standard features are that it does not occur in both sexes, women being not affected, that it comes about from exsiccation, and that it involves the anterior part of the scalp, especially the region about the coronal commissure. Thus Galen wrote that alopecia, ophiasis, and calvities attack the head and the beard, a statement to be interpreted disjunctively, not conjunctively (the head and/or the beard).

It may be asked why, if calvities affects all men merely because of age, I should call it a disease rather than something that is natural. It seems that the disorder occurs not simply from natural causes, but that indeed nature intends that it should occur. I reply that calvities, however naturally it occurs, nevertheless goes beyond the purposes of nature. There are several reasons. First, it sometimes occurs prematurely. Furthermore, it is contrary to the tendency of nature to generate hair on the head. Galen wrote that adornment and comeliness are the purposes of nature in generating hair, whereas, when the head is deprived of it, the adornment and pulchritude intended by nature are denied. Thus the ancients when they went bare-headed were anxious to hide their baldness, as if calvities were a shameful defect.

As to the cause of calvities, there is controversy among the authorities. Hippocrates seemed to think that warmth is a factor. This particular reference is suspect, or at least whoever wrote it managed to misuse the meaning of "calvities." We think the writer was perhaps someone other than Hippocrates himself. Elsewhere

Hippocrates wrote that calvities is brought about by depletion of the brain. In discussing this, Galen said that as a man's age progresses the brain withdraws from the cranium so that the bone, deprived of moisture, can no longer sustain the growth of hair, which, lacking nutrition, dies and falls out.

Aristotle, the greatest of the philosophers, gave another explanation when he wrote that calvities comes about because of inadequate warmth and moisture of the fat, which therefore becomes cold and dry. Aristotle was quite reasonable in saying that fat is moist and warm and that, when a man starts to grow old, the outer moisture becomes increasingly watery and cold. The moist, warm fat disappears, as John the Grammarian and Averroes explained, because it exists by virtue of digestion, which is impaired in old men so that this kind of moisture cannot be generated.

Galen appears to have attributed the disorder to only one cause, drying out alone. I agree with Galen that dryness is one factor. While recognizing the non-functioning of moisture as another cause, as Aristotle stated, nevertheless I cannot say that Aristotle was the more discerning. A certain modern author, however, errs when he would censure Galen for saying calvities is due to dryness, then offers the explanation that bald men do not sleep. For sure this is fabulous. Even if the brain is dry in old men for lack of moisture and so of fat, yet actually excrementary moisture is increased in them, and the brain is continually moistened by the wetness of their food, so they do sleep.

The antecedent primary (procatarctic) causes of calvities are all those that are capable of drying out the brain: insomnia, worry, late study, and immoderate coitus.

Alexander suggested that calvities is in fact transmitted by heredity, as gout is.

The diagnostic features (signa) of calvities are in brief as follows. It begins in the frontal region and progresses gradually. It comes with age, and, furthermore, it occurs at the time of becoming capable of coitus, as Aristotle said when he observed that eunuchs do not become bald, nor do boys prior to puberty. In the absence of other causes of defluvium, calvities is indicated. The preeminent feature, however, is that when remedies are applied that are effective for regenerating hair, it is nevertheless not generated.

Galen and Aristotle gave but one prognosis: true calvities is incurable. However, medical effort can retard it in its early stages.

At this point six intriguing (fine) problems are involved, well worthy of consideration. First, why does man alone among all creatures develop calvities? While, as some say, the ostrich and certain coots known as "phalakrokarakas" grow bald, this is not true calvities. Metaphorically, even trees are said to become bald, as by Columella. The second problem is why is calvities irreparable despite all medical endeavor? The third is why do some grow bald quickly and others slowly? Galen stated that the Ethiopians become bald the slowest. The fourth is why do women not grow bald? Both Hippocrates and Galen concur that they do not. Indeed, Synesius the Philosopher, in his book on calvities, specified that from time immemorial women with calvities have never been seen, but Albertus Magnus stated that he had seen two cases. The fifth problem is why does calvities start at the front of the head rather than at the back? The sixth and final problem is why are bald men the descendants of bald men, as Hippocrates and Alexander both attested?

With regard to the first problem, Aristotle wrote that only man becomes bald because the brain is larger and more humid. Averroes, however, said that only man becomes bald because he alone has capilli. Some may disagree with Aristotle, arguing that, if calvities results from inadequacy of moist fat, it would seem that man, with the most moisture, should not be subject to the disorder. John the Grammarian, seeing the difficulty, called attention to the fact that man's brain is the coldest, and he felt that this should substantiate Aristotle's description, so as to mean that man alone becomes bald because his brain is the wettest, largest, and coldest. It is as a result of coldness that heat subsides and moisture and warmth waste away.

This explanation seems inadequate because creatures in their infancy are actually subjected to extreme cooling and so should be subject to the condition. I am thus obliged to argue that man does not become bald solely through the influence of an extremely cold or wet brain but rather because he alone has capilli, as Averroes said. The fur (pili) of beasts, since the constituent hairs are extremely coarse, is not dependent on moist, warm fat and is more easily retained on that account. Man has capilli that are fragile and fine, readily liable to injurious influences.

I may be asked why has nature not provided man with pile that is tough and not prone to shedding? And why, if calvities is injurious to health, should not nature show greater concern for our welfare than for that of beasts? I reply as Plato did with regard to the structure of the whole human head. The natural plan is that the human head should be effective in both bodily health and mental function. If nature wished the hair of the head to be durable, man would surely have been incapable of mental activity. Hence nature chose a balanced constitution that does not interfere with either bodily or mental functions. Furthermore, man, being imbued with rationality, has been able to compensate his want of pile with some sort of covering. The philosophical Synesius put it cleverly: "Prudence and pili are incompatible." Thus it is that the hairiest creatures, sheep for example, are the stupidest (imprudentissima), while those with few hairs, man for example, are the wisest (prudentissima).

The second problem is why calvities cannot be cured. Aristotle argued that, as the foliage of trees is renewed annually, so is the hair of animals. This bodily change is seasonal, spring, autumn, winter, and summer. As the seasons are annually recurrent, so are the changes in creatures. Strictly speaking, man changes in accordance with his ages (life stages). Because these do not recur, his vicissitudes (mutationes) of the hair are, as is true in other matters, not renewed.

A further explanation can be adduced. The evident deficiency of moisture in calvities is irreparable because the fat and warm moisture imparted to man at birth, although conserved by virtue of the digestion, nevertheless diminishes daily and cannot be replaced while heat is progressively deficient and the energy of digestion weakens. This explains why Galen said that some people become bald: they have had a dry brain since birth, and an even drier scalp.

With regard to the third problem, the physician Cassius explained that some grow bald more slowly, others more quickly, because some men are warmer than others. He added that those who are of a cold temperament are unable to sustain the capilli. He would seem to say that those who become bald more gradually are the warmer. In my opinion, this is unproven. We have seen that calvities is brought about by the lack of moist warm fat, and it necessarily follows that those who are too warm would become bald more quickly because moisture is used up most rapidly by the greatest warmth, whereupon calvities would develop. Thus we must agree with Galen that those who are late and slow in becoming bald are those whose brain is of moderate temperature, and those who become bald early are the ones with dry brains.

Alexander said that individuals with curly hair lose their hair sooner because they have a drier brain. We must take special note of this passage, being hesitant as to whether the fault lies in dryness of the brain or dryness of the skin. Dryness of the skin does not always predispose to calvities. Indeed, Galen wrote that, just as trees, although taking root with greater difficulty in hard soil, yet, having become rooted, remain for a longer time; so also it is more difficult for hair to grow on a dry skin, but when it has grown, it lasts longer and falls out less readily. This is the reason, according to Galen, why the Ethiopians, although their hair is of a loose texture, nevertheless become bald less frequently than other peoples.

As to the fourth problem, Aristotle explained that women do not grow bald, just as boys do not, since they do not produce semen. Long ago the medical profession rejected this belief, for many believed that women and boys too make semen and emit it. In support of this idea, there is a statement of Hippocrates to the effect that boys before the age of fourteen do have semen but do not emit it because the vasa (deferentia) are too narrow to provide a passageway. So it must be said, with Galen, that women and eunuchs do not become bald because they are of a cold temperament, and their innate heat cannot destroy moist fat, which persists enduringly as nutrient for their hair.

We can offer yet another explanation. The fact is that women's heads have fewer sutures. Of course moisture is preserved in the brain for a longer time in individuals with fewer sutures. As Hippocrates wrote, men with no sutures have the wettest brains. This may explain why the Ethiopians do not become bald, if it is true, as Arrianus wrote, that their heads lack sutures. So it must be concluded that women do not become bald because they are of a cold temperament and have extremely wet brains. As Averroes put it, women do not become bald because of their moist complexion.

As to the fifth problem, why calvities begins at the front of the head rather than the back, Aristotle explained that the most vigorous part of the brain is contained there. To clarify this opinion, Averroes said that calvities involves this region simply because it is thinner and warmer than other parts and therefore moisture is the sooner used up, and so calvities develops. Substantiating this view is the fact that in infancy the front of the head is the softest. The same explanation may be given as to why calvities involves no other part of the body. Alexander said it involves the frontal scalp because that region is lax and so is deficient in nutrient, and the hair falls out, and this does not occur in back because the skin there is firmer and denser, and this permits less hair loss.

As to the sixth and last problem, I should say that calvities is not hereditary in the way gout is. But what have we to say about the opinions of Hippocrates and Alexander? Hippocrates wrote that individuals with large heads (macrokephales) are descended from individuals with large heads, and those with gray eyes from gray-eyed parents, and bald men from bald fathers (calvos ex calvis). Alexander was of the same opinion, so it appears that my view conflicts with theirs. I say Hippocrates and I are both correct. I am, I say, because I speak of true calvities, while Hippocrates in the passage quoted did not. He spoke, rather, about those who throughout life are hairless, whose disease he inappropriately called calvities. Heroditus, Strabo, and Pliny told of a certain people, of Mikonos (one of the Cyclades Islands in the Aegean Sea), and certain others, of India, who all their lives are without hair on the head. It is of this condition Hippocrates spoke, not of true calvities.

About the cure of the condition, I have nothing to say, for once established it is absolutely incurable. But I will speak of preservation of the hair, which a physician is obligated to know about, for two reasons. First, whether one becomes bald quickly or slowly is pertinent to the preservation of health. Secondly, most people consider baldness disgraceful in a young man, many of whom therefore beg a physician for remedies for its prevention.

Now it may be asked how the lack of hair can be detrimental to health. Galen wrote that hair may actually be injurious, especially in conjunctivitis (ophthalmia) and nasal catarrh. Synesius the Philosopher recounted many cases of ocular affections and catarrh cured solely by cutting the hair from the scalp. Some say the Egyptians depicted Aesculapius as bald so that doctors might be taught by their preceptors that calvities contributes to good health. While in some situations and in some individuals calvities might be beneficial, I should say that for the most part and in most cases the loss of hair is detrimental to health, for it would allow drafts to penetrate into the brain, actually harming it.

As for preservation of the hair, there are two objectives. The first is to retain and conserve as long as possible the moist warm fat whereby hair is nourished. The second is to bring about a condensation of the skin in order to keep hair from falling.

Toward accomplishing the first objective, the diet is of paramount importance, and one recommends foods such that those that promote dryness are avoided. The best nutrients are fatty and rich foods of a kind that nevertheless can be utilized to good effect. Fruits are apt to considerably accelerate calvities because they provide moist, flimsy (flaccidum), unsubstantial nutrition on which hair could not thrive and would readily fall out.

Temperate air is to be preferred, cool rather than warm. To avoid calvities it is wise to wear a hat to prevent the injurious effect of the air. Loss of sleep is very bad, and worries, too. The sole explanation in many a case of calvities is too little sleep and too much worry. Indeed another cause is too frequent coitus, which hastens baldness, and the patient should refrain from sexual excess. Combing and rubbing the head too frequently hasten baldness, and those who would avoid it must beware. An excess of wines and strong drink is apt to cause baldness by a drying process. Alexander in discussing the devotees of Bacchus said that many who follow him become bald from the harm the brain sustains from intemperance.

Toward achieving the second objective of condensing the skin, one must apply scalp lotions as well as certain inunctions. The lotions should incorporate the agents that strengthen the skin and condense it. Whatever they may be, they must not conduce to the wasting of moisture and fat.

Take the extract of 10 pounds of grapevine ash, 6 pounds of bitter red wine, 2 handfuls each of madder, rose, and plantain leaves, and 2 handfuls each of green nut shells, pomegranate shells, and myrtle. Boil together until a fifth part is consumed. Then wash the head once a week with warm cloths, avoiding excessive friction. The lotion should not be too hot.

In conjunction with the wash, certain liniments should be used to counteract the smell the inunction may produce. Oil of labdanum mixed with myrtle juice and green nut shell juice will be the most useful. One can be made, for example, as follows. Take 1½ ounces of distilled oil of labdanum, ½ ounce each of myrtle leaf juice and green nut shell juice, 2 drams of finely pulverized or liquid mastic, and 3 grams of amber. Mix and make a liniment. The front of the head could be anointed with this daily.

It is important to note that cutting the hair frequently right down to the surface of the skin contributes greatly to the prevention of baldness, for not only are the remedies more easily applied, but also, since short hairs cannot consume much nourishment, the moist fat by which the capilli are nourished is conserved. Therefore, above all else, one should shave the hair frequently right down to the skin surface to prevent calvities.

On this subject Heroditus wrote that the fewest bald heads were seen among the Egyptians because they habitually shaved the scalp, with the result that the skin was made firmer and thicker.

Galen listed many other remedies for the prevention of calvities, among others that of Andromachus the Younger, the one called "pericalamitis" (adarce), which Galen said his friend Claudianus used in curing two cases of true calvities.

Such remedies can be continued as long as we desire. I will not give their descriptions, which in Galen's works are available to anyone.

BOOK ONE, CHAPTER SIX

ON CANITIES

OF THE DISEASES of the capilli, Galen listed canities last. While not detrimental to the body, yet it is of importance to the physician. Galen wrote that two aspects of the hair, comeliness and elegance, are of medical concern, but in different ways. Comeliness, concerned as it is with the preservation of natural beauty, rightly falls within the province of medicine, while elegance of appearance, although conducive to a polished and artificial beauty, does not; yet, as Galen said, it must be recognized by the physician on account of the fashions of women of dignity. I do think that the study and treatment of canities, if undertaken primarily for the preservation of natural pulchritude, fall in the first category.

Canities is called "poliosis" by the Greeks. Thus Homer, as we are told by Alexander, spoke of the patients as "poliokrotaphoi," i.e. white-templed. The condition was described in a book of Galen's as premature whitening of the hair. One must recognize that what is called simple whiteness (albedo) of the hair and canities are quite different.

Canities is of two types. One is that which occurs in the course of aging, and the other, that which Aristotle recognized as being clearly related to defects and diseases. Galen included this type within the category of vitiligo. Avicenna called it the canities of youth. We shall discuss both types.

First, let us look into the causes of the canities of aging. On this subject medical authorities have various opinions. Some of the old writers thought it due to dryness, saying that, as we see the leaves of trees dry up and become white and hoary, so we see that hair when it dries up becomes white. Aristotle proved this wrong on two counts. First, those who go about with the hair covered become white-haired more quickly than those who go bareheaded, yet the latter are dried out quicker. Since the former develop canities less quickly, it must not be due to dryness. Secondly, there are many whose whiteness of the hair begins at the time of birth, when the body is patently most moist. Ctesias pointed out that, in a certain race in India, women bear children only once, and the infants as soon as exposed to light immediately begin to show white hair. Thus, as Aristotle wrote, canities cannot come from dryness.

Here is a matter on which I do not wish to remain silent. I have repeatedly called attention to the fact that Athenaeus attributed erroneously to Aristotle what he himself wished to say, that canities comes from dryness. Furthermore, one may not ignore the fact that, when Aristotle showed that canities does not come from dryness, he did not insist that it might not come about in some other way. As Averroes made clear in his commentary on this passage, dryness is simply incidental to canities. I would say that when hair suffers in the course of an illness or some other cause, its moisture and viscosity are diminished so that its root (substance) comes out shiny, even transparent.

Jacobus, my fellow citizen, in his commentary on Galen adduces another explanation of how dryness may be related to canities. Its dark, moist substance emerges and dries, and this is what blackens hair. As the blackness (pigment) disappears, the dark color recedes, and whiteness becomes apparent.

The great Hippocrates seems to have held the opinion that phlegmatic moisture, over a protracted period of time, imparts a finer and whiter character to the hair, which, when so nourished, becomes white. This is the reason, he added, why people with blond hair have blond skin. Avienna seems to have accepted Hippocrates' opinion, as apparently Alexander did too, but Averroes (under, however, an assumed name) refuted this on the basis of his view that the hair is fed by an ultimate nutrient that is not phlegm, but when hair is nourished by phlegm—so he said—it is so altered as to be unable to hold its color.

Aristotle had a different idea, in many ways better than the others', when he wrote that canities comes about through an inadequacy of innate heat, which is therefore unavailable to the humors, so that the hair, lacking it, is attacked by external heat, hence becomes decadent and eventually white. The reason why hair whitens from decadence is that the humor as it decays is to a great extent changed into air (see gas), and this, mixed with earthy and watery substances, brings about the white color, as was clearly explained by Aristotle. The same explanation, said Averroes, applies to the whiteness of butter, camphor, and foam.

Galen, following Aristotle, said that canities comes from phlegm decadent because moisture is scanty and viscid. For want of heat it decays easily.

Here one clearly recognizes that Galen borrowed the idea from Aristotle, who said that canities is "tina eurota," a kind of decay, or actually a decayed vapor, just as phlegm, a white substance, is a condensed emanation (vapor); for Aristotle wrote that the Comics called canities "eurota," decay and hoar-frost.

Thus the views of Aristotle and Galen were the same as to the cause of the canities of old age. It is evident that Avicenna, although in other respects a most reliable author, erred when he imputed to Aristotle the idea that canities represents a conversion to the color of phlegm. The whiteness of the hair, as Galen taught, does come from the whiteness of phlegm, but the idea that phlegm causes canities was nowhere stated by either Aristotle or Galen.

Pertinent to this speculation, four brief questions come up that deserve consideration. One is, why does canities begin at the temples? Another, why do men and horses as well grow white with age? Thirdly, why do women develop canities faster than men? Finally, why does canities appear more quickly on covered heads than on bare?

As to the first question, Aristotle's explanation was that the moisture about the temples is of such a quantity and kind that many people cannot resist its decay in the region of the sinciput, whereas the quantity is so scanty at the occiput that the moisture can be heated more easily. He apparently meant that the moisture in the temporal region decays more easily than in other regions of the head, and therefore canities begins more quickly there. Galen, following Aristotle, explained that the temporal region becomes white with age first because it is more moist, and he went on to explain that the excess is due to the presence of large muscles, which are moist because they are fleshy, and make the whole region moist. Artistotle and Averroes added another reason. The bones of the temporal region are so thin that external heat enters easily, and this sets the corruption going. Evidence that these bones are thin is the fact that wounds in this location are deadlier.

To the second question one must reply that man most of all becomes white-haired because he of all creatures remains the most moist. Aristotle explained that horses become white with age because they have thin bones. I believe, however, that the humor in them decays easily because the animals are of a cold nature. To tell the truth, we ought to say that these conditions are not true calvities but represent simply whiteness (albedo) of the hair.

As to the third question, why women become white-haired with age more quickly than men, the same reason applies. They are of a cold and moist nature and so more susceptible to corruption. If canities is brought on by corruption, as has been said, it makes sense to find that women should become white more quickly. On the other hand, people with black and curly hair, being of a drier nature, become white more slowly; and those with red hair, more quickly.

As to the fourth and last question, the reason why those who cover the head become white-haired more quickly is because the natural heat of the head is unable to get out, stifled, as it were, and held in by the hair. Thus, it is that when natural heat is lost in a short time, the humors, deprived of it, decay easily. This explains why frequent applications of ointment hastens the whitening of the hair, not because they dry it out, as was argued by Athenaeus, but because the passageways of the head are so obstructed that they cannot let vapors out (exhalare).

Whiteness of the hair that may be called "canities morbosa" is of two kinds, that which follows vitiligo and that which follows any other disease. Canities secondary to vitiligo develops simply because in vitiligo the skin becomes white from vitiated nutrition, and its hair so nourished necessarily becomes white too. This is how Avicenna's statement must be interpreted when he wrote that canities results because the blood becomes watery.

The canities secondary to other diseases results solely from corruption of the humors and their consequent albescence.

When hair is nourished by corrupt and white humors, it becomes white, as we have said, and this is why many people become white-haired suddenly from fright or grief. Those who become white-haired overnight have been heard of frequently, and many authors have recorded such reports.

What is to be said about distinguishing canities due to age from canities secondary to disease? Four signs are diagnostic of canities of old age. The age characteristically is either ripe old age or early senility. The canities develops slowly, not suddenly. It starts at the temples, and it actually involves, according to Aristotle, the ends of the hairs, for the tips are weaker, as Aristotle and Averroes both noted.

The diagnosis of canities secondary to vitiligo is made from the color of the entire body. How vitiligo comes about I will elucidate in the proper place. Canities due to other diseases may be recognized first by the fact that it comes on not slowly but suddenly, even in a few days. It may occur in youth. The whole head becomes white at the same time. Later, after the primary disease has begun to subside, the hair darkens again.

The canities of old age presages nothing but old age itself. It is thought by common folk to be a bad omen, but by prudent men to be a rather good one, as we see in Plato's works. Every kind of canities resulting from disease is bad because it indicates a serious lack of natural heat and a great abundance of moisture.

Let us now discuss the treatment. Canities secondary to vitiligo is treated by the same measures as vitiligo, and this we will discuss in the proper place. Canities arising from another disease is cured only by such means as are effective for that particular disease. Aristotle said that secondary canities is eliminated when the primary disease is. Nonetheless, certain precautions must be observed, especially as to the diet, and these, if strictly observed, will greatly help to hasten the cure.

Among the beneficial measures are massage of the scalp, frequently combing, and exercises for the whole body. These will strengthen the natural heat and actually open the pores of the scalp and, consequently, tend to abate the corruption of the humors and so to do away with the condition.

Rhazes wrote of a friend who got entirely rid of white hair by taking 1 dram of chalcanthite, or vitriol, every evening. I know this remedy has been highly recommended by many physicians, but Galen's advice has pleased me. He condemned the use of chalcanthite as an oral medicine. ("Chalcanthite," derived from Gr "flowers of bronze," inexplicitly used in ancient times for blue vitriol, copper sulfate, and for green vitriol, iron sulfate, also known as copperas. We may imagine that Rhazes gave iron sulfate with favorable effect while Galen gave copper sulfate and wished he hadn't.)

Canities due to grief, anxiety, or other passions of the mind is easily cured if all the causes of such problems are eradicated. Canities that comes about through age and lasts until life ends is incurable, all physicians agree. Even in such cases, however, two kinds of remedies are available. One might retard the process if it is still in its early stage, and the other, although not curative, nonetheless can darken the hair and perhaps mask the color completely.

The following are remedies for blackening the hair. While Galen said that canities is neither disgraceful nor damaging, nevertheless men and women are sometimes so importunate in hounding the physician that familiarity with the treatment cannot be ignored. Some of the measures for retarding canities have to do with food, others with medication. Those who would postpone canities should be especially vigilant regarding food and should avoid warm, thick air; for as we have said canities comes about through decay induced by external heat. Moderate exercises help a good deal, as does massaging the head and the whole body, and also combing; and one must take special care not to cover the head at all. One must see to it that the bowels are kept loose and regular, and that all perturbations of the mind, especially anxiety and grief, be dispelled.

On the subject of food and drink Rhazes wrote that one should abstain from rich, heavy wine. All dairy products should be avoided, and, furthermore, fruits, fish, oils, and legumes. Foods to be chosen are those that are easily digested and nourish optimally. In Rhazes' opinion, fried and roasted foods are preferable to boiled. Beneficial are pepper and small amounts of mustard, cinnamon, and any other aromatics customarily sprinkled on the food.

Effort should be made to avoid indigestion. Avicenna put it nicely, saying that digestion is at the root, as it were, of all therapy, while indigestion is the cause of almost all bodily ills, as Galen had noted in his booklet on foods.

Then, too, there are medications for external use and for taking internally. If we would follow Aristotle, external medication ought to be cold for counteracting the warmth of the external air, but only moderately so, however. The skin pores should not be occluded. Thus Aristotle approved oil and water for keeping the pores open. Going farther than Aristotle, Galen taught that external medication should be heat-inducing and mildly exsiccative. This is not unreasonable, since the major goals in preventing canities are the restraint of decay and the elimination of whatever has been corrupted.

Medicines of this sort are the ones that are warming, exsiccative, and penetrant by reason of their fine texture. In this class, cedria is the preeminent choice. Galen recommended many other things, such as leech dung mixed with ox gall and ashes of the verbascum white blossoms and colocynth pulp steeped in vinegar, the last highly praised by Oribasius, Johannitius, and many others. All Greek and Arabic authors praised oil of the wild olive and cypress nut plasters applied to the scalp, along with the internal use of myrobalan, which many think will retard the development of canities if frequently applied. The same is true of baths taken while the stomach is empty. Rhazes recommended scalp lotions containing colocynth, salt, and ox gall. In using these lotions, he particularly cautioned that the head must be dried completely and carefully after washing. Marcellus, hardly unworthy as a physician, recommended washing the scalp with a decoction of pure white lamb's head. Such are the things that help to retard the progress of canities when applied externally.

A number of external applications ought not to be used. First, Rufus of Ephesis taught that scalp lotions made of plain warm water should be avoided. We know the great difference between using warm water or cold when one wishes to wash clothes white. Cold water darkens them, and warm water whitens. Rhazes was of the opinion that rose water is outstanding.

Plucking the hair frequently should be avoided, although a good many people do it. Hippiatrists (horse doctors) who wish to make white spots on horses pluck the hair frequently, following which, it has been observed, they may grow back white. Rhazes rightly condemned excessive bloodletting. Avicenna especially cautioned those who wish to avoid canities to keep their hair from coming in contact with sambucine oil, camphor, and plain water.

Many internal medicines for this condition deserve commendation. Among them, those that drive out phlegm and serous humors are thought to be especially suitable. Pills properly made of agaric, if taken over a long period of time, cleanse the body of phlegm and do no harm. Confection of anacarda, theriac, and mithridate are among the remedies to be taken internally to protect one from canities. Avicenna especially recommended frequently chewing East Indies myrobalan and eating snake meat, which in the opinion of physicians from antiquity contributes more than anything else to the preservation of youth.

Among the Arabs there was a certain mixture for retarding canities that is praised to this day. It is made as follows. Take 40 drams of pitted black myrobalan and 10 drams each of ginger and bishop's weed (ammi). Moisten with butter and add taffy to make up about a half of the total. Taking a dram or two of this confection frequently is recognized as perhaps the best remedy for preventing canities.

Other medicines, the ones that blacken hair, do not prevent the whiteness, but do hide it. This treatise is concerned with the more dignified arts, but, as we have said, Galen cautioned physicians not to neglect the subject, for vain white-haired women, anxious not to displease their husbands, often insist on remedies of this sort.

The art of dyeing hair was introduced into Rome not until after the time of Heracles of Tarentum (160-110 B.C.). Up to Galen's time (130-200 A.D.) it was held in such esteem that some men did not blush at dyeing their own hair and actually wore wigs.

The coloring agents are, as Galen taught, bitter, astringent, and cold. They have often proven to be the source of serious diseases in women, apoplexy, epilepsy, catarrh—a veritable Iliad of maladies. It is always best to avoid strong medicines of this sort and adhere to those that are less hazardous, such as cedria, which Galen said he used only in the cooler and more moist conditions. In other cases correction and improvement are obtained with simple oils.

In Galen's day, there were medicaments containing oil and pitch for restoring black hair. Those most highly recommended were acacia, nutgalls, fenugreek, hyocyamus seeds, dried coriander, spikenard, labdanum, green nut shell juice, poppy juice, iron rust, chalcanthite, black comfrey (alumen), and burned copper. Various scalp locations were made of these, and they are still in use and popular in liniments and lotions for darkening hair, also a lotion of black myrobalan, ox gall, and myrtle.

Two things should be noted about these medicines. They do no good unless they are used over a long period of time, and one should not be disappointed if they do not work within the first or even the third day. As Galen warned, they should not be given to everyone who asks, but only to patients in whom good results may be expected. This is the place to say that one may have to omit cedria and pisselaeum (pine tar) because they smell so bad.

As I tell some women, there is one particular agent that always darkens white hair within a month or less. Take 1 ounce of black myrobalan, 2 ounces of dark raisins, and 3 pounds of dark astringent wine. Boil in a double boiler over a slow fire until two-thirds is consumed. Add the juice of 5 pounds of green nut shells and 1 ounce each of sumac and acacia, 1½ ounces of cariophyllus leaves, and 1 scruple of musk. Put this on the stove again and, without boiling over, keep it hot for half a day. This will darken the hair without danger of injuring the scalp. One thing I must emphasize as to its use. It should be painted on the white hair with a brush at bedtime, and the head should be bandaged overnight. The next morning wash the head with dark, astringent wine in which black myrobalan has been boiled.

I could give many other formulas, but they can be found easily in the literature, and we must hasten to the consideration of more important matters. So I bring my essay on disorders of the hair to an end and begin the discussion of diseases of the scalp.

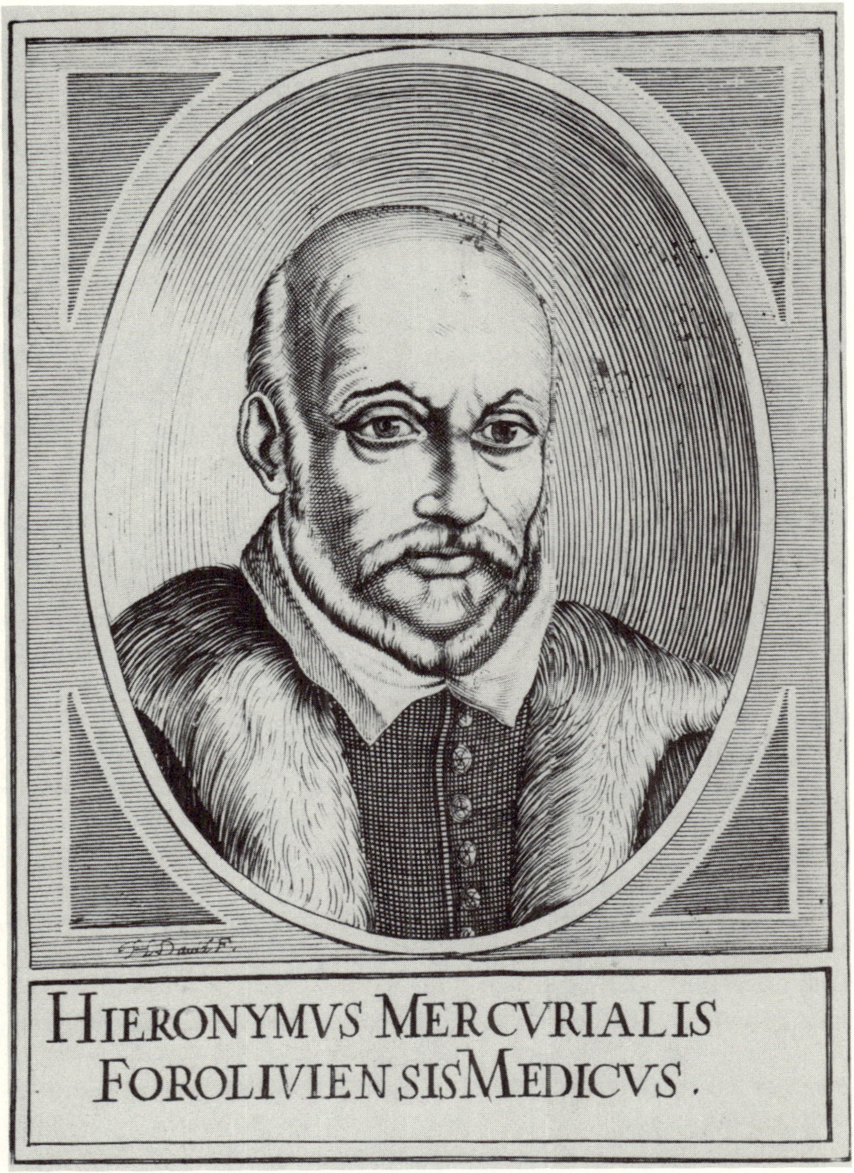

This illustration was published by "Thomasinus: Illustrium Virorum Elogia," Iconibus Exornata, Padua, 1630, Donatum Pasquarum et Soc. A photograph of the original in the collections of the Forli Institute of Arts and Culture was provided by Dr. Walter Vichi. The artist was David Heronymus, who was born in Paris in 1605 and died in Rome about 1670. His likeness of Mercurialis, who died in 1606, must have been created by the artist or copied from an unknown source.

BOOK ONE, CHAPTER SEVEN

ON PEDICULOSIS

THERE ARE some diseases of the scalp with ulceration (? exudation), others without. The nonulcerative diseases are called "pediculation" and "furfuration" (the lousy and the scurfy). The ulcerative diseases are achors and ceria, or favus, which Aetius and Celsus called "meliceris" (honeycomb lesions). Among the ulcerative diseases are sycosis and psydracium (vesiculopustular dermatitis, from Gr psydrakion, blister), all of which we must discuss.

We will start with the conditions that are not ulcerous, and first with pediculosis, called by the Greeks "phthiriasis" (Gr phtheir, louse), therefore known as "phtheiriasis" and spoken of as "apo ton phtheron" (from lice). This is the derivation Galen gives.

This disease arises from corruption of the humors and is one in which lice are generated particularly on the head. I say it is a disease, because it is an unnatural condition that harms the functions of the body. It interferes with sleep, as we shall show, and is to be classified with the type of diseases that include the intestinal worms. While we are speaking primarily of the scalp condition, lice are produced all over the body, a matter we shall discuss; but they originate on the head.

As to the generation and causes of this disease, there are various views. Aristotle was of the opinion that lice come from corrupt flesh, and he made three points. First, in infested patients there is a preliminary formation of pustules which, when they discharge, yield lice. Secondly, he said, the condition affects individuals with extremely moist bodies, or develops after certain diseases. Thirdly, birds, fishes, and all quadrupeds suffer this kind of disease, except the ass.

Aristotle's views do not seem to me completely valid, for two reasons. First, lice are produced in the scalp, where the flesh is thinnest. If they came from corrupted flesh, then surely youngsters' heads, which swarm with the evil animals, would be completely consumed. Secondly, lice abound in the second and third varieties of fevers, but in these the flesh is so consumed that no place would remain for lice to be generated. Thus there is no way for lice to reproduce from corrupt flesh in the manner Aristotle proposed.

Theophrastus had a different explanation, suggesting that lice come from corrupted and decayed blood. To me this does not seem true, for two reasons. First, in fevers in which blood does undergo decay, there is no apparent production of lice as evidenced by any indication of corrupt blood within the materia of the lice. Secondly, since origins attest to their principles (ultimate sources), if lice were actually derived from blood, some of them should appear red and bloody, but such are not seen. The fact is, the color of lice is quite different from that of blood, and it is plain that they are not generated from corrupted blood.

We have next to verify the explanation given by Galen and Avicenna. Lice come from the warm excrements of the third and final digestion, decayed but neither irritating nor perverted (pravus). To make this interpretation fully intelligible, we must realize that when blood is converted into the substance of the body members, many kinds of excrement are produced, some of them undergoing dissolution through insensible evaporation, others through the sweat, some being converted into sordes, and still others, retained in the skin. If they are retained in the superfices of the skin, they induce scaling. If they are retained deeply in the skin, either they are defective and irritating and so produce ophiasis, or they are not, in which case they produce lice. Thus lice originate from the warm excrements of ultimate digestion, not irritant, not deformed (? pathological), but wholesome (dulcibus). Such is the material cause of lice.

We see that the efficient cause of lice must be heat, as all authors seem to agree, but what is uncertain is what kind of heat. Avicenna seemed to think that two kinds of heat work together to bring this about. The one is cosmic and may be called creative or "chol-codeum," the other, particular, which he called "natural." The former would be the mediate cause, the latter, the immediate.

This theory raises two questions. The first is how natural heat can generate anything in decayed stuff, which if actually decayed is devoid of natural heat as long as the process of decay is dominant. The second is whether this view of the generation of lice is correct, seeing that lice, as Aristotle said, actually infest fishes.

As to the first question, some say the sense of Avicenna's opinion should be taken in the negative, that he meant an unnatural heat gives rise to lice, an explanation I consider fanciful. Others say that the heat of decomposition is of two kinds. One decomposes materia perfectly and completely, consuming it wholly, and the other corrupts materia only imperfectly, not destroying it totally. The former, they say, is incapable of generation, but the latter brings about generation by decomposing materia incompletely. Since the materia is not completely decayed, it is rearranged in a different configuration so as to take the form of life.

This interpretation does not seem tenable to me. While the heat of the decaying does not completely corrupt the materia, nonetheless, since it is extraneous and is of the nature of decay, it is quite unable to dispose materia for taking up the living form, a property limited to natural heat itself. Then, too, this explanation cannot agree with the statement of Avicenna, who said that the efficient cause of lice is natural heat. But this heat is indeed not natural, so I must repeat what Aristotle said when he discussed those things that come from decayed materia. He wrote that decay of itself cannot produce anything, but that everything is generated by concoction (digestion involving heat). We infer from these words that, in Aristotle's opinion, when anything is generated from decomposed matter, generation may actually occur, but concoction is also always involved. If there is always some concoction, then necessarily, in all such generation, there will be innate heat, because concoction is the property of innate heat alone. I say therefore that every decay from which something is generated involves a residuum of natural heat that is not completely destroyed but imparts to the thing digested in a proper and orderly manner the disposition to live and assume a bodily form.

This must be true of lice. They are concocted by natural heat when it digests the moiety of the humors that is decayed.

With regard to the second question I reply that the lice that infest fishes do not come from the fishes themselves. They are not of the same genus (descent, origin). Aristotle says that the lice that harass and torment fish are generated in slime.

With regard to the final cause, Quintus Serenus held the view that nature creates lice to interrupt sleep so people may stay awake at night and get their work done. The following verse is quite apropos:

> Noxious substances from our own substance nature
> engenders, to interrupt slumber, admonish the senses,
> and wakefulness, too, for giving mind to our cares.

This idea deserves to be exploded, I think, especially as it applies to pediculosis in the young, who need sleep. If nature really intended this, the effect would be damaging. I confess that those who live on ships may need lice to keep them alert, but children don't.

If any final cause for lice can be given, one may believe with Avicenna that the decayed humors in the body are used up in the process, or that, as Averroes said, lice exist so that nature should not be idle. For sure, nature would hardly take a holiday but may be expected to be always productive of something. In the generation of lice and of other creatures, nature seems to have no purpose but to express its restlessness.

As to the site of generation, Avenzoar agreed with Galen that lice are procreated in a median location between the skin and the flesh (subcutaneous tissues). If one would concur with Aristotle, one may, on the authority of Avenzoar, interpret him to mean that lice are not generated out of corrupted flesh, but rather in a place between the flesh and the skin. The truth, according to Avicenna and Galen, is that the site of generation is deep in the skin.

Many predisposing causes of this disease are listed by the authorities. First are age and indeed sex, for Aristotle wrote that women and children are affected particularly. Children especially, but also men, are sometimes infested with pediculosis of not only the scalp but also the whole body, sometimes of such severity as to prove fatal. Aristotle referred to such a death in the cases of Pherecydes, the Syrian, and Alkman, the poet.

Galen wrote that eating papaya strongly fosters the growth of lice. A change of water, the omission of exercise, uncleanliness, and negligence in the care of the body and in the changing of garments, especially the underclothing, are conducive to pediculosis. Thus prisoners and sailors are often afflicted, for they seldom wash.

Close association with a case of pediculosis is the main factor in producing the disease. Even light rubbing of the head, said Avicenna, produces lice in great quantities. Correctly understood, he did not mean that rubbing the scalp will produce the disease if the body is clean; rather, if the disease is present, then even light massage will promote it by increasing the warmth—not by introducing lice, but by making conditions favorable for their generation. It is in this way, Avicenna said, that coitus with an unclean individual causes the disease. Eating snake meat will greatly augment the production of lice in those whose bodies are already infected, as Galen taught.

Many varieties of the affection are listed by various authors. Some pediculi have many feet and perambulate from place to place, and are called hexapods by some authors (? body lice). Others lack feet and are not ambulatory but remain fixed, permanently eating away. Aristotle called them "agris" (ferox) because they are harder and more difficult to extract from the skin (? ticks). Then there are those commonly called plactulas ("little flat ones," ? pubic lice). Some lice will grow but little and stay on top of the skin, walking about with agility nonetheless and irritating, and these are popularly known as pedicelli ("the ones with little feet," ? body lice). Others, equally small, remain on the hair and are called lendines ("little smooth ones," fr L lenis: ? nits). While there are various differences between lice, they all come of one materia.

The characteristic features of the condition I shall not describe, for they are self-evident, but I will say something about diagnosis. Aristotle wrote that all who have head lice have heads that are quite healthy in other respects, the explanation being that in both their reproduction and feeding the animals use up a great amount of excrement, so when freed of this the head continues to be healthy in other respects.

Appolonius said it was Aristotle who observed that in moribund patients lice abandon the head and are to be found on the bedding. Explaining this, Alexander said that lice abandon a person who is about to die because they require warmth and fresh bloody liquid. When these juices are not available, it is easy to understand, the lice leave to seek better places.

This disease is entirely bad and evil, particularly when it increases in severity, for, as we have said, it is not only degrading but also disgusting, sometimes even fatal. These animals are generated in the early stages of lepra and in the second and third species of hectic fevers.

Since the disease is one to be dreaded, every effort should be made to learn its cure. It represents an abnormality of the humors, of which some already exists and some is being produced, so that two objectives are apparent. The first is to prevent increment of the humoral abnormality, the second, to remove the extant abnormal humor. This is continually accumulating through nutritional errors, so the primary need is a dietary regimen such as will not promote decay. Although Galen and the other Greeks were silent as to the dietary aspect, yet it is indeed not to be neglected.

As Galen wrote, there is nothing effectual in the way of benefit, nothing that can be productive, unless done in conjunction with a dietary regimen. First, one must carefully avoid eating to excess, omitting harsh foods and injurious juices. The meats permitted are birds, such as doves, chickens, and the like. Some authorities are opposed to pheasants, which are especially subject to pediculosis, as if eating their meat would transmit the disease. Papaya especially is frowned upon by all authorities because it does what Galen said snake meat will do, that is, if taken frequently, it is apt to promote the generation of lice. Avenzoar, a great physician, recommended cooking meats and all other foods in vinegar, omphacium, or barberry juice. We need not be concerned with what to drink, because wine is quite equivalent to water.

One must be much concerned with exercise and physical fitness. The patient should undoubtedly exercise before eating. Just as inactivity promotes this disease, so exercise carries it away. Bathing regularly before dining is advisable, but baths after meals are harmful. One must painstakingly keep the body clean and remove wastes daily. Patients must be attentive to changes of clothing, particularly the underclothes. Certain kinds of clothing have been shown by experience to considerably promote the generation of lice, especially the wool from dead and putrid sheep. I emphasize this because doctors must guard against it.

When this regimen has been established, we proceed to the purgation of humors already decayed. The intestinal tract should be cleansed with any mild preparation. The following is appropriate. Take 1 dram of diacatholicon and 2 drams of electuary Ind. Mix and make a bolus.

After the intestine has quieted down, we come to medication for the humors. Since great corruption has entered the blood, the first procedure is bloodletting, as much as the body can tolerate, from the left side unless strongly contraindicated. Syrups are meanwhile prescribed to prepare the humors. Take, for example, 1 handful each of borage leaves, tormentil, scabiosa, and pedicular herbs.

Make a decoction in the usual way. Then take ½ ounce of this decoction and add 1 ounce each of syrup of scordium and of syrup of lupine. Mix and make a draught. Whoever takes this syrup for 7 to 9 days will believe he is getting better.

The humors thus prepared should be drawn out with great care, and for this purpose a number of medicines have been praised by Avicenna and Avenzoar, including agaric, carthamus, and hiera of iron. Galen thought highly of his aloes pills. Thus the following medication might be prepared. Take 1 dram of the best agaric, 1½ drams of carthamus, 1 ounce of raisins, and 1 scruple each of ginger and cinnamon. Infuse in goat's milk whey, letting it stand overnight in the usual manner. When the material has been expressed carefully, add 3 drams of Hamech's confection and 3 ounces of violet honey. Mix.

If it is more appropriate to use pills, we have the aloes pill Galen liked. We might use pills of agaric or hiera with colocynth. If these do not work well and the patient does not respond promptly, one may consider repeating the purge. Really this ought to be done, because if anything can remove the disease, expulsive and repeated purgation can.

After purifying the body, we come to the medicines that will eliminate the abnormal humors embedded in the skin and are capable of correcting the distemper of the body. Some are to be given internally, others applied externally. The internal medications, according to Avicenna, are boiled allium and mountain-grown calamint. Mustard was recommended by Paullus and Serenus. Theriac is a medicine likely to be helpful, and powdered staghorn is excellent.

External medicines, Galen taught, should be exsiccative so as to gradually consume all decay, and finely particulate so as to penetrate the innermost recesses. Medicines of this sort are saltpeter and staphisagria, which was called "uva taminia" (lit. cluster of wild grapes) by Galen, the louseherb by others. Hellebore is an excellent medicine, as is sandarac, according to the Greeks.

These are reduced to a fine powder and put up in an ointment.

If they prove too mild to eliminate the disease completely, we come to those that are stronger, among which the most potent is quicksilver, a dangerous medicine, not to be used casually. The following is a formula for it. Take ½ dram of quicksilver diluted with saliva, add 1 dram of sulfur, 1½ drams of powdered burned staghorn, and vinegar and oil q.s. to make a liniment. This is suitable, as we have said, in extreme cases, not to be used unless the body has been purged most completely.

Paullus, Aetius, and others strongly recommended washing the head with a decoction of wormwood, lupine, rue, abrotanum, and salt. These are all highly commendable because of their bitterness, exsiccative power, cleansing ability, and abstersive property.

In some cases women, and perhaps men who have been weakened by prolonged illness, are infested by lice, particularly of the head, but cannot tolerate overzealous treatment. Here is the formula I usually use in extreme cases, a formula that does kill lice but is without harmful effects. Take 1 small handful of staphisagria and 2 drams of saltpeter. Boil in 4 pounds of water until half is consumed, express, and add 1 dram of diluted quicksilver. Stir with a stick for 2 hours. Wash the scalp with the liquid, and apply it under a cap. Then wash the head, and dry. If the patient's scalp is wrapped in this way, for some reason the animals will die after a day or two, and the patient will be cured.

Theodorus Priscianus thought well of cedria, a resin from the cedar tree, a substance said to have caused strangling when taken internally. Applied externally, it will keep bodies from decay and corruption. Quintus Serenus thought well of bran steeped in vinegar, but this is a mild remedy, useful only in early stages of the disease.

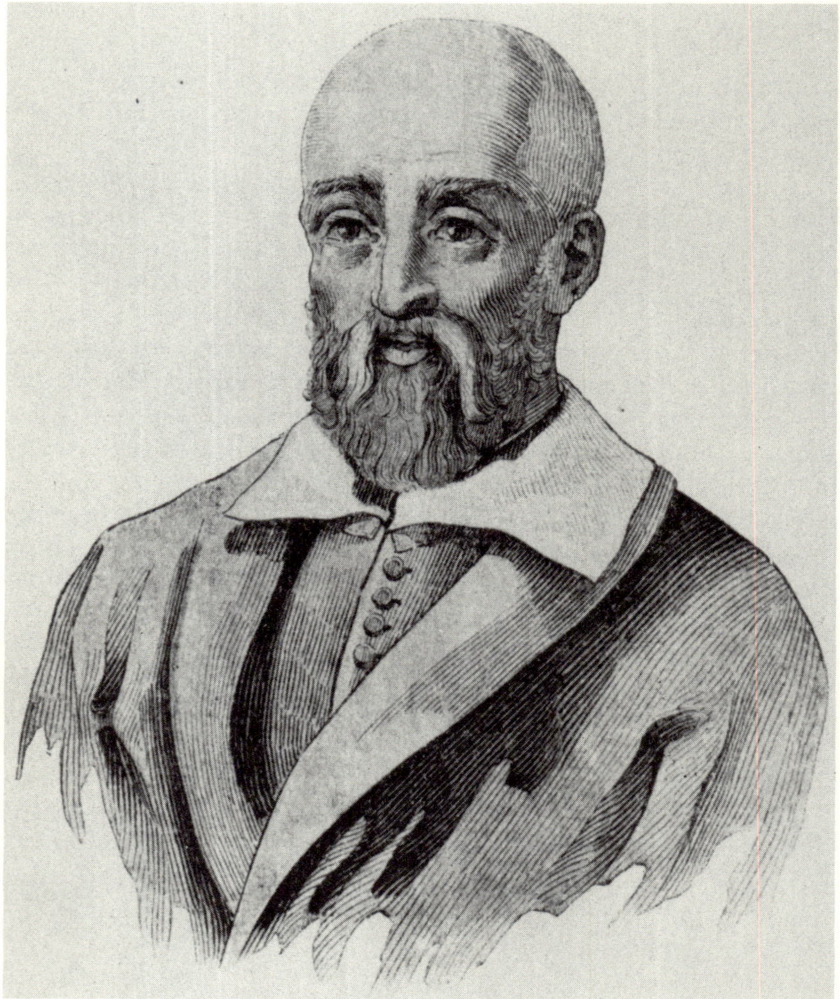

GEROLAMO MERCURIALE
1530-1606

This illustration was published on the front cover of Romagna Med. Nov. 1956 by Busacchi, V., et al., an issue dedicated to the memory of Gerolamo Mercuriale. It was a copy, done toward the end of the nineteenth century, of the original published in Forli in 1835 by Antonio Hercolami in his "Biographies and Portraits of Illustrious Figures from Romagna," vol. 1, p. 23, with drawings done by F. Spagnoli and engraved by Hercolami. This information was provided by Dr. Walter Vichi of the Forli Institute of Arts and Culture.

It was used also by author(s) of the article in Chirurgia degli Organi di Movemento vol. 2, fasc. 3-4, pages 259-274 (Aug.) 1918.

BOOK ONE, CHAPTER EIGHT

ON PORRIGO

RELATED to pediculosis is a different disease called "pityriasis" by the Greeks, "porrigo" by Cornelius Celsus and the Latin writers, and "furfuratio" by foreigners (? seborrheic dermatitis). It is a common and distressing disease. It appears in the form of scales and flakes seen when the head is scratched, as Galen taught. Paullus added that it may involve any part, or the entirety, of the body, with or without sores.

Cornelius Celsus, describing the development of the disease, said it appears about the hair in the form of scales, sometimes moist but more often dry. As it appears, it may or may not be exudative (ulcerative), sometimes malodorous, sometimes not. The scales frequently involve the head, rarely the beard, sometimes the eyebrows.

Paullus and Cornelius Celsus, both authoritative, nevertheless expressed contradictory views. The former thought that the disease never involves the whole body and that it is sometimes ulcerative. The latter, however, said that it does sometimes involve the whole body and occurs only in a nonulcerative form. Quintus Serenus was of the view that it involves only the head, as the following verse indicates:

> The disease, without symptoms, in appearance is noxious; furthermore, from the scalp on combing, the scales seem to snow a profusion of flakes, as if from a flour mill.

Galen was apparently of the same opinion.

To eliminate contradiction, we refer to Avicenna, who wrote that porrigo is of three varieties. It may be of the kind that involves essentially the head, recent or of long duration, or that kind which accompanies a defective state of the whole body. With this distinction in mind, it is easy to reconcile our illustrious authorities. When Paullus said that the disease may involve the whole body, sometimes with ulceration, he was speaking of all the varieties, not only the chronic cases involving the head, but also the acute kind and the kind that is concomitant. When Cornelius Celsus said it involves only the scalp, beard, and eyebrows, he was leaving out the concomitant type and speaking only of the varieties, chronic and acute, that essentially involve the scalp. In his discussion of the subject Avicenna said that furfuration is sometimes so severe that it may even become ulcerative so as to destroy the hair. We should say, with Alexander, that furfuration is generally, but not always, nonulcerative.

As to the immediate causes of this affection, Galen was of the opinion that it is generated by corrupted ichors. Some have gotten the impression from Galen that there is a difference in materia between porrigo and lice. They have said that the materia of pediculosis is thick and viscid, while that which generates furfuration is thin and ichorous. Unanimously opposed to this view were Paullus, Alexander, and Avicenna, who all agreed that the disease is generated from materia that is phlegmatic, salty, bilious, and melancholic when it reaches the head. Avenzoar said that it comes from salty and defective phlegm.

It is clear, according to our most illustrious authors, that the disease is not always brought about by thin humors but may come from dense ones. But what shall we say of Galen's authoritative views? I think that by defective, corrupted ichors Galen actually meant humors that are defective, corrupted, and also thick, for it is the universal practice of writers to speak of the humors in this way. Galen's opinion in this matter can be inferred. He contrasted the humors that disperse strongly from those that are detersive. It is clear that the medication for thick humors is no less appropriate for thin ones.

There is another significant uncertainty as to whether this disease may actually be due to a distemper (intemperies) of the head. On the one hand is the view of Galen that I cited and of Paullus and all the Arabs, who said the disease comes from morbid humors. Alexander of Tralles said it comes from defective body juices (cacochimia), a passage misunderstood by Nicolaus of Florence. On the other hand, there is the authority of Galen himself, who wrote that porrigo may come from a distemper of the head alone, adding that the body juices are all right. Galen taught, it is quite clear, that porrigo is due simply to a distemper of the head.

This questionable point is clarified by the words of Avicenna, who wrote that porrigo sometimes comes from corrupt humors that reach the head in corrupted form and sometimes from humors that reach the head healthy but undergo corruption there. It is our belief that porrigo comes invariably from corrupted humors and that, whatever may cause the trouble, it cannot occur unless the humors are defective. As for Galen, it must be said that his view of porrigo as being due to a distemper of only the head must be interpreted as meaning that sometimes sound humors are transported from the body into the head and are there vitiated and corrupted so as to make porrigo. He did not mean that these humors are in the head or the body, but that they are corrupted in the head as a result of the distemper there.

What Galen's opinion was can easily be understood. He was refuting the interpreters of Hippocrates, who were correct in saying that Hippocrates connected porrigo with breathing, but the view that breathing pushes deformed humors from the body into the head, Galen said, is not so. The presence of porrigo is not due to the rising of deformed humors from the body into the head. In conclusion, we say that in porrigo, deformed humors must necessarily be present, and a distemper of the head is not of itself a sufficient cause.

In addition to the material and immediate causes of porrigo, there are other factors which, while not actual causes, nevertheless contribute considerably to the production of the disease. Factors of this kind are frequent overeating and taking salty and acrid foods, such as salted meats and fish, onions, garlic, and the like. Excessive coitus and unsuitable or inappropriate exercise before meals are in the same category. They all abet the development of the condition. So, too, do baths, either cold or warm, when taken after meals.

The features by which the disease is recognized are quite apparent. Small flakes that fall from the head on mere rubbing or light combing are a clear indication of its presence. Which humor causes it one can tell from the color of the skin. If it is red when the scales have been removed, sanguine materia is evident; if yellow, bilious; if bluish-black, melancholic; if whitish or nearly white, the humor is mucous and phlegmatic.

The cure of this condition differs little from that of pediculosis, for in each the materia is the same, undoubtedly a corruption of the humors. The objectives of treatment are apparent. First, the decay must not be allowed to spread, and secondly the decadent humors in the body must be removed. If a mere distemper is present, without the humors, this should itself be corrected and eliminated.

To achieve the first aim, establishing a good diet is a dependable measure, so reliable that, as Galen and we ourselves have said, it alone suffices to cure many cases, even the stubborn ones. The patient must abstain from salty, acrid dishes and rich and harmful juices and should drink either plain water or thin, weak, white wine. Avenzoar objected to plain water and thought it should always be mixed with honey or boiled wine. His advice ought to be followed, for, as we shall show, the disease originates from phlegm.

Archigenes, as quoted by Galen, strongly favored establishing a dietary regimen for the condition. He wished especially, and not without reason, to permit no foods that make gas and no thick and harmful juices. He particularly objected to onions, legumes, and tubers, for which in an ancient version of his text sorb was substituted by that ancient interpreter (Galen), who thought the text corrupt. Mushrooms were condemned also, but he recommended foods with good juices and those easy to digest. For a sauce he recommended vinegar with sape. He thought well of fennel and cumin. These foods are most effective for exsiccating a condition of decay, so he would have the patient abstain from fruits and pastries, but of these raisins and figs are best and may be enjoyed in preference to the others.

Morning and evening walks before meals are quite helpful in this condition. For washing either the whole body or the head, especially in the summertime, cold water is recommended and hot water enjoined. One must forbear anger. If anything increases suffering in this disease, it is fits of anger that make the humors boil. Immoderate coitus is a factor that makes the disease worse.

When this regimen has been established, one should consider whether the basic defect is in the whole body, in some particular internal part, or in the head alone. If it is in the whole body, one must attend to this first; likewise, if it is in an internal organ, one must devise the appropriate cure. As for bloodletting, Paullus, Alexander, and Avicenna were of the opinion that this should always be done when the defect involves the whole body. Whether the defect is in the whole body or in some particular viscus, one is obliged, I think, to consider whether bloodletting might be harmful. It might be done more than once if indications of overabundance were present. If it is a distemper of only the head that harms its juices, bloodletting would, however, be omitted, and one might leave off the purgation of the humors and start local measures immediately.

First the flakes should be removed from the head with light massage or gentle rubbing. When the scalp has been cleansed, it should be washed with a mixture such as one that contains equal parts of decoctions of mallow, althaea, rape leaves, and beet leaves. Instead of soap, ground bitter almonds are good for taking off and drying up all kinds of scurf as well as for strengthening the skin.

After the scalp has been washed and the flakes rubbed away, one must still combat the distemper of the scalp that has been brought about by heat, and this necessitates the use of some kind of cooling inunction such as rose or lilac oil, nenuphar, gourd oil, or any other that cools the skin and checks its fever.

If the faulty state involves the entire body, one must determine the particular humors that have been corrupted and are aggravating the disease. If they are phlegmatic, one must treat them with medicines appropriate for expelling them from the body, not just once or twice but again and again. If they are bilious, one must do the same, and this is true of melancholic humors, too. I omit giving here instructions as to the methods of preparing the humors and purging them, for I listed all of them when I described the management of alopecia and ophiasis, to which one may refer (Book 1, Chapter 4).

If blood has not been let, we might use a small cupping glass with multiple scarification, which will readily remove the vitiated blood dispersed in the skin.

After the body has been purged, we take up local measures. As to their use, we must consider whether medicines for strengthening the skin are appropriate. They would appear to be suitable in cases where there is an influx of materia. The medical precept, not to be ignored, is that in every kind of influx the recipient part should be strengthened. On the other hand, on the authority of Cornelius Celsus, a most learned physician, this is a condition in which the skin should not be strengthened. His reasons are cogent. Nature made the skin the weakest part of our body to serve as a receptacle for corrupted humors, hence the physician should not interfere with this natural process, for if the vitiating humors were not purged by the skin, those retained might easily harm the nobler parts.

As to this perplexity, I should say a physician can strengthen the skin in two ways, either to a slight degree or to a considerable degree. The latter is precluded largely for the reasons Celsus gave. For sure in this condition the skin should not be greatly strengthened, but it may be strengthened a little, as Galen believed, and all the Greeks, and even Celsus, himself, as evidenced by the fact that he did not shrink from using mild astringents, such as myrtle wine. Galen, following Archigenes, was not content with myrtle wine but used more efficient astringents such as vitriol (atramentum sutorium, lit shoemaker's black).

The views of Archigenes and Galen must be interpreted as applicable to chronic and stubborn furfuraceous diseases. Avicenna distinguished three varieties, one mild, one moderately severe, and one severe and ulcerative. He advised that the mild type be treated without bloodletting or purgation, using gentle measures only. We have already described the way it should be treated in considering the management of mere excessive scaling of the scalp. He recommended the use of stronger medication in the more severe type and extremely strong medicines in the most severe. For cases of the second category he liked the abstergent and moderately loosening ones. Both he and Galen suggested many of this kind, such as fenugreek, beet leaves, bitter almond, pumice, myrobalan, wild mallow, staphisagria, incense, and cimolia. These were recommended by Paullus. From them one can prepare powders, liniments, and lotions.

If a powder is appropriate, it may be made as follows. Take 2 ounces each of fenugreek and dried beet leaves and 2½ ounces each of black myrobalan and staphisagria. Pound and reduce to powder. The right time for the powder is after the head has been massaged and prior to washing. The powder should be applied to the scalp and rubbed rather briskly with the hands. Then the head should be washed with the following decoction. Take 1 handful each of beet leaves, staphisagria, and mallow root. Boil in 8 pounds of ordinary water and add 1 pound of mildly astringent white wine. Ground bitter almonds or pumice, ground or whole, should be used in place of soap, as I have already advised.

If a liniment of these ingredients is desired, it may be prepared as follows. Take 3 drams each of beet leaves and powdered black myrobalan, white myrobalan, and staphisagria, 2 ounces each of ordinary oil and myrtle oil, and 1½ ounces of vinegar. Mix.

Make a liniment.

Heretofore we have shown what medicines are appropriate for the second type of furfuration. It remains to be seen what is appropriate for the third type, which is the most severe and requires the strongest medicines of all. Many such were listed by Galen and Avicenna, including saltpeter, sulfur, colocynth pulp, veratrum, chalcanthite, ox gall, and various grain meals, such as those of lupine, beans, or barley. Liniments and lotions can be prepared with these ingredients.

Powders are prepared as follows. Take 2 drams each of saltpeter and sulfur, 1½ drams of colocynth pulp, 1 dram of black hellebore, and 1 ounce of roughly ground lupine. Mix, pulverizing carefully. After shaving the head, as we have said, rub this in briskly.

In place of soap, the scalp lotion should contain roughly ground lupine and barley. Latin authors called the rough grain "farra" (a mashlike fodder in contrast to "farina," a meal or flour, and "farrago," a mixture of grain, a mash).

A lotion is made as follows. Take 1 handful each of beet leaves and althaea root, and 2 drams each of colocynth pulp, white hellebore, and saltpeter. Tie these up in a bundle and boil along with the herbs and roots in 10 pounds of water until one-fifth part is consumed. Add 2 pounds of white wine, and use this to wash the head.

If the disease is still obstinate and the sores unyielding, use the following ointment. Take 1½ drams each of blue vitriol and ox gall, 2 drams each of saltpeter and sulfur, and 2 ounces of rose-scented omphacine oil. Mix over a fire in a double boiler and make up an ointment with a small amount of beeswax.

This is the way to cure the more severe furfurations that respond poorly to gentler medicines.

Cornelius Celsus thought the head should be shaved frequently and smeared with some mild astringent. He thought highly of myrtle wine with labdanum and, too, myrobalan with wine. These medicines are helpful only in mild and moderately severe cases, not in the chronic ones. When the scaling is moist, Paullus recommended scalp lotions made of strong salt water or sea water, or from a decoction of lupine. Alexander of Tralles recommended these too, saying he had tried them with considerable satisfaction and found them quite helpful.

BOOK ONE, CHAPTER NINE

ON ACHOR AND FAVUS

HERETOFORE we have discussed the scalp conditions without ulceration. We shall now discuss those that produce ulcers when they affect the scalp, all the affections that many of the Arabian school, Haly Abbas in particular, called "tineas." Avicenna and Serapion called the disease "sahafati" in their language and said that it occurs not only on the scalp but also on the face and body. Theodorus Priscianus wrote an account of it.

We shall divide our discussion into two parts, following Avicenna. The first will be concerned with the scalp ulcers the Latins call moist, or "manantia" (exudative fr manare, to drip). Common folk speak of them as "milk sores" (ulcera lactumia). Various names are used by the peoples of various countries. The second part of my discussion will be concerned with the dry sores called tinea (L worm) by many physicians and known as such even by the laity today. These are common diseases of man, so knowledge of them may not be disregarded.

Beginning with the moist sores, let us see just what achor is. Alexander of Tralles and Julius Pollux used the word as if it were "ichor." So with no unkind feeling I say of Cornarius, otherwise a learned physician, that he was in error in his commentaries on Galen when he said something different (from Galen) about this name. Achors are actually tumors of the scalp in which openings appear from which exude thin, rather sticky humors, as Galen, Oribasius, and Aetius have said. Paullus of Aegina would say a sticky humor. Theodorus Priscianus said the achors are "papillas" (little nipples), unless one would call them "papules," which emit an extremely oily humor through cavities that are quite short and are frequently located on the head, face, and other parts.

Quite similar to achors are certain other moist ulcers that Galen called "kerta," and many Latin physicians termed "favi." Theodorus called them "kerion;" Aetius, "meliceris." Other authors, including Paullus and Oribasius, used Galen's nomenclature.

The difference is that the openings are smaller in achor, larger in favus. Alexander of Tralles drew another distinction. In achor the openings are not visible, while in favus they are. Theodorus Priscianus, too, described the differences. In achor, strictly speaking, there is one opening of one cavity, and from this a thin humor exudes; in favus, however, many cavities are present, and a thicker humor comes from the lesions. On one point, however, all authors agree: the humor from favus lesions resembles honey in consistency, so that meliceris and kerion are appropriate names. Rhazes said that favus is a crusted form of tinea (tinea crustosa) from which exudes an evil humor that resembles honey from a comb.

Two kinds of moist and exudative ulcers, then, involve the scalp, the one called achor, the other, favus. Both were apparently called meliceris by Cornelius Celsus, although there are many errors in the chapter I quote, errors which have, however, been corrected in the latest text; but the manuscript codex gave "kerion" for "meliceris." These two kinds of sores first begin with intense pruritus, from which swelling develops when it is scratched, and this enlarges daily; and a humor oozes from it, sometimes thick, sometimes thin.

To avoid error, we must note that, while Aetius and others called favus meliceris, meliceris is a different type of tumor wherein the materia occurs in little pockets, and this does not occur in either achor or favus.

The material cause of this affection, according to Galen, is an acrid, serous, erosive humor mixed with a thick one. Avenzoar, deviating from Galen's view, said the ulcers come from an acrid, bilious humor accompanied by one with some thickness. Paullus of Aegina seems to have considered the material cause phlegmatic, nitrous, and salty. One notes that he spoke of them in two places but did not describe two types, since it was one and the same disease in both descriptions. In his third book he spoke of them as disorders of the scalp, and in his fourth, as abnormal swellings. That the conditions were not different is indicated by his reference in his fourth book to what he said in his third. Alexander of Tralles wrote that the ulcers sometimes come from phlegm, sometimes from bile, and occasionally from melancholy. These authors can be reconciled with Galen, for the nitrous and salty phlegm Paullus talked about consisted of bilious, acrid, irritating, and phlegmatic liquids. His view did not differ from that of Galen, nor did Alexander's, since by definition these ulcers, both the moist and the dry, were included. Avicenna averred that the dry ulcers come from a melancholic humor, and this we shall explain at the proper place.

As to the mediate causes of these sores, Marcellus the Physician considered age a factor, and noted that childhood is the time when one is particularly susceptible, but that men and women are too, even more severely and with greater damage. The explanation of the susceptibility of children to this disease is that while in utero they are filled with excrements that nature intends to expel soon after birth. The greater part is expelled through the head because, of all the parts of the body, the head is the most moist and the fullest.

The disease reaches children from the mother's milk. Perhaps nursing women, because of their insatiable appetites and poor selection of foods, suffer a deficiency of juices, so that their milk is infective and communicates the defect to the children. Other causes are the improper food and drink men and women are likely to ingest. Thus the disease comes through a contagion, as is apparent from the fact that nurses become infected by the children they nurse.

A special proclivity for the development of these diseases occurs in certain geographic regions. I recall a physician from Sulmona who wrote me for information as to the cause and cure of these diseases in those regions. The time of year appertains, for Avicenna recorded the fact that the ulcers are most frequent in the winter.

The diagnostic features are evident, partly from observation and partly from the history (relatione). In both conditions considerable pruritus is usually present at the onset, following which the tumor develops and apertures appear, and from these liquid exudes, sometimes watery, sometimes thicker. In some instances lice are present. Rhazes thought it particularly characteristic in favus for scales to be present around the sores, but actually this feature is common to all cases. When the scales are removed, the materia of each kind of ulcer is recognizable.

The color, as Paullus taught, is diagnostically informative. If it is pallid, the case abounds in bile; if white, in phlegm. Alexander of Tralles said that other diagnostic features are recognizable, such as the temperature of the patient, his age, the taste, and the feel. As for the taste, if this is slightly bitter, it is an indication that the case comes from bile; if acid, from acid phlegm or melancholy. Similarly, from the feel: if the ulcer is somewhat warm, this indicates that the materia generating the disease is bilious; if cold, phlegmatic.

As for prognosis, these sores in common terminate in defluvium, as a rule, the severity of which varies with the degree to which the materia is abnormal. Thus the sores may possibly extend and progress not merely into alopecia but into ophiasis and exulceration of the flesh and even the bone, particularly in advanced cases. Hippocrates wrote that, if the sores occur in the scalp, about the ears, the face, or even the rest of the body in a child, it may be cured of the epilepsy, an observation confirmed by Avicenna.

As to the cure of these conditions, we must first recognize that, since the disease usually involves children, medicines are to be used in minimum quantities, especially internal medicines, for two reasons. First, it is unsuitable for children to take drugs. Secondly, mothers fear, not without reason, that these may injure their children's health, so they are themselves reluctant for them to be treated. When physicians are obliged to medicate patients of tender age, Rhazes advised that, if the infant is suckling, the nurse must receive attention. She must avoid deficient juices (pravi succi), bitter and salty foods, milk, fish, and eggs that have been baked or fried. She should omit wine and avoid venery, and finally she must avoid everything that generates thick and defective humors. Milk immediately assumes the qualities of what has been eaten, and since infants are nourished entirely from it, of necessity they drink in all of its qualities.

Beware of portulaca, for this has the peculiar faculty of making the disease worse, Avenzoar warned. According to Galen, Archigenes objected even to the use of vinegar.

When the regimen has been instituted, we turn next to local medication, but we again mention the recognized fact that a nursing woman ought to be purged, and this should be done before she uses local medication. If she is bilious, one should use agents appropriate for purging bile; if phlegmatic, those for eliminating phlegm.

In discussing local medication, Alexander of Tralles seems to have taught that it should be of a repellant and astringent nature. Alexander was apparently referring to adolescents rather than small children, for such medicines are quite dangerous in the very young. Their scalps are especially full of humors. One should conform with Avicenna, who proposed mildly astringent topical medication capable of moderate exsiccation, such as indigo together with roasted nutgalls and the fat of a ram's tail. For example, take 1 dram of indigo, 2 drams of roasted nutgalls, and ½ ounce of ram's tail fat. Mix and make a liniment. Avicenna said that this is the best medicine he ever tried, the one in his own experience most advantageous. He also suggested pomegranate bark, with vinegar, oil of roses, and litharge, and he spoke highly of massage with vinegar and salt. It must be kept in mind that most children are to be treated with mild medicines. I say this because vinegar and salt massages are excruciatingly painful. Further, Avicenna suggested tutty, cimolian earth, burned paper with vinegar, and bitter almonds.

I will now tell you about two medicines I use, usually with great success. One is for the youngest children, the other for those fairly well grown. The first consists of the following. Take 1 dram each of myrtle ashes and nutgalls, 1½ drams of tutty, and 1 ounce each of lotion of rancid butter and rose water. The ashes are levigated with vinegar, then mixed over a fire. The other medicine is made up as follows. Take 1½ drams each of powdered pomegranate bark, litharge, and tutty, ½ ounce of oil of roses, and 1½ ounces of goose grease washed with vinegar. Mix and make a liniment.

In using these, one should remember two things, one as to the method of their use, the other as to the fats. First, the unguent should be spread with soft brushes previously dipped in wax. Brushes so dipped keep the heat of the sores from using up the medicine. Furthermore, a tight-fitting cap thoroughly smeared with medication should be kept on the head constantly because children often tear the medicines off.

The second point to be remembered concerns the fats. When we wish to use them for exsiccation, we should choose the ones that are aged because, as Galen wrote, these possess discutient and exsiccative properties. On the other hand when we desire an emollient effect, we should always use fresh fats. One must note that while old fats tend to exsiccate more effectively, they tend also to become stronger and hotter with the passage of time. It is not safe to use exsiccative agents alone unless the heat of the ulcers and their acuteness are blunted thoroughly. One must wash these fats off repeatedly, as many as five times. Washing, particularly with vinegar, removes the irritant quality due to the age and the heat too, increasing the exsiccative effect rather than diminishing it. Rose water will wash away butter and fats as may be necessary.

On the subject of fats, I will resolve a nice contradiction in Galen's writings, one which, as far as I know, no one else has noticed. Galen wrote that goat fat is extremely irritating and fiery. Elsewhere he said that there are ways to prevent pain. One may eliminate salty things and the like, or one may relieve pain by applying such things as pure olive oil, barley oil, and goat fat. It looks as if Galen contradicted himself, for in the one citation he said goat fat relieves pain by tempering it, while elsewhere he spoke of this grease as acrid and fiery.

To dispose of the contradiction, two points occur to me. The first is whether the goat fat is recent or old. Old fat is especially acrid and hot, as Galen mentioned, while new fat, although irritating, is not so much so as old, and Galen mentioned this. Thus new fat is advantageous. It does irritate briefly but nevertheless has greater ability to soothe than to irritate, and this is why Galen recommended it.

I am not fully satisfied with this explanation. In the passage I quote, Galen appears to have meant that goat fat is quite irritant as long as it is fresh. I have thought that the passage might be corrupt and that it should read "aigos" in place of "tragou." I came to this conclusion because Galen said that in the treatment of dysentery the fat of the mountain goat is valuable. It is much less acrid than ram fat because, taken from about the intestines, it not only ameliorates pain but prevents further mordication (corrosion).

So far we have discussed the management of achor and favus in children. It remains to be seen what should be done for adults, for mature individuals are frequently attacked, as the Greeks and Arabs all agree. On the subject of treatment they said the first thing to do is to institute a proper dietary regimen, the principal features of which have been established: the avoidance of excessive food and drink, the selection of nutrient of the best juices, and the avoidance of rich wine, sweet, bitter, salty, and fried foods, and all foods that evoke thick and bitter humors.

After this diet has been instituted, we consider the purging of the defective humors. First, one must decide whether, along with the defect of the juices, there may be a superabundance of blood, and, if indications of this are apparent, beyond doubt blood should be let. If the head is extensively involved, Avicenna advised that the head veins, the frontal or the postauricular, be incised, and if the disease affects the whole body, the veins of the feet should be opened, according to Avicenna or, in our opinion, the vena communis (the common ulnar vein). The amount to be withdrawn is in proportion to the body habitus.

After venisection comes the purging of the humors, which are to be prepared by the following syrup. Take 1 ounce each of oxisaccara (sugar and vinegar), syrup of lupine juice, and syrup of borage juice, and 1½ ounces each of the aqueous extract of borage, lupine, and scabiosa. After this has been prepared, the patient should be purged with an agent for eliminating sluggish and thick humors. If the medicine is to be given in pill form, pills of hiera Pacchius may be prescribed or pills of agaric with alandahal troches. One may make a bolus of the following. Take ½ ounce of rose sugar, 2½ scruples each of rhubarb and finely pulverized agaric, and 6 grains of lozenges of violets and scammony. Mix. Make a bolus, to be taken in the morning.

A draught good for purging the humors is as follows. Take 1 dram each of choice agaric and rhubarb. Make an infusion in the usual way with the whey of goat's milk. Take 5 ounces of this and add 3 ounces of syrup of polypody, or of Hamech's confection, and 2 ounces of dilute rose syrup.

After good purgation, we turn to local medicines, in the choice of which one must first consider whether the disease is in an early stage or is chronic. In the early stage, Alexander rightly advised that we must use astringent and repellent agents. Suitable for this purpose are rubus leaves, salix, plantain, juice of oleaster, myrtle, pitch-pine bark, and polygony. One makes a lavacre (bath) of these or an ointment for the head. The bath is prepared as follows. Take 10 pounds of chalybeate water and ½ pound of willow leaf ashes. Lixiviate (leach) and add with boiling a small bundle of leaves of the red rubia, 1½ handfuls of plantain leaves, and ½ handful each of myrtle and pitch-pine bark. Boil, strain, then wash the head.

After washing and drying, the following liniment may be applied. Take 1 ounce each of rose-scented omphacium and oil of myrtle, 2 drams each of juicy myrtle leaves and oleaster leaves, and 1 dram each of red rubia powder and myrtle powder. Mix and make a liniment.

If the disease is in its early stage but complications threaten, Archigenes, according to Galen, advised that an astringent agent should be added to those that are moderately exsiccative. One of this sort is made up by mixing cyperum, lentils, and labdanum with myrtle oil and a small amount of wine.

If the disease is chronic, one must consider whether the sores are mild and superficial or severe and deep. If mild, Galen said that they can be cured by a dietary regimen alone, short of evacuating the body. But even in these cases local medication is often necessary. Agents are chosen that are able to attack, penetrate, attenuate, and exsiccate, such as vinegar, which has these properties. Some metallic medicines steeped in vinegar may be applied, such as the following. Take 2 drams each of tutty and spodium, 4 drams of litharage, ½ ounce of rose-scented omphacium, 2 ounces of vinegar, and beeswax sufficient to make a soft liniment. Mix. If it is rather soft, it is all right.

If the disease does not yield to these remedies, something stronger must be used. Among such are lime, ashed lees of wine, sandarac, quicklime, and burned conch shell. Such medicines are potent exsiccants, good for drying up and curing chronic and stubborn achors. In these cases the head should be washed vigorously with the following mixture. Take 10 pounds of chalybeate water and ½ pound of fig wood ashes. Leach. In this boil 2 handfuls each of leaves of sharp lapathum and beet roots. Strain the decoction, then wash the head.

After washing and drying the head, the following preparation is best. Take 2 drams of ashed lees of wine, 3 drams of lime steeped in vinegar, ½ ounce of burned conch shell, and enough old oil to make a liniment.

While these are most effective, one must keep in mind the fact that they are potent and more suitable for sturdy patients than weak ones. Then, too, as Galen said, some achors are quite painful, inflamed, and angry and must be treated differently. In these one must apply medicines that soothe the pain and assuage the raw humors, the agents that moisten, soften, and soothe. The one most praised by all writers is called "pharugron" (iron rust), also prescribed by Paullus. If this is not available, one may substitute a cataplasm (poultice) of finely ground lentils and honey or of wheat flour and green coriander juice, or even of plantain juice, or of polygony juice with finely ground barley or wheat. These are more or less alleviating, softening, and drying.

If the pain is relieved by this kind of medication, the head may be washed with a decoction of fenugreek or beets, especially recommended by Galen and others because it softens raw achors moderately and dries them somewhat. A number of other medicines recommended by Apollonius and Crito were listed by Galen, who considered fenugreek and beets best.

More recent medical writers have thought that a class of diseases should be established that is neither achor nor favus, but between them. In justification of their view they quote Galen and Rabbi Moses (Maimonides). I examined the references carefully and found that these writers were mistaken. Although Galen said that achor comes from materia that may be thin or thick, favus comes from a thicker one, and he insisted that no achor consists of thin materia only. So we might say that a type of disease derived from delicate and coarse humors might constitute a middle group.

We now come to the plan of treatment of achor and favus, the same in children as in adults, and on this subject there are some considerations worth noting. First, in treating these cases the hair should not be plucked but merely shaved or cut, for the hairs are not much corrupted unless the achor or favus is of long standing, in which case they frequently are. When the hairs are not corrupt, they should merely be shaved. If this is not done, the medicine cannot be helpful or effectual.

Another point to be noted is that Galen recommended a preparation of paper ashes for chronic and recalcitrant sores. He said that when he was living in the country, paper ashes steeped in vinegar cured these cases in a remarkably short time. Descriptions were given in the works of Galen and of Paullus. If all the authorities thought so highly of this remedy, we should like to know if it is available to us now. Of course, we do not have the paper of the ancients. Pliny is the only source of information as to how it was manufactured. There were two ways, from papyrus steeped in the waters of the Nile, or from papyrus so prepared and then mixed with glue, but I do not wish to take time examining Pliny's description.

Papyrus is a kind of rush that grows profusely along the Nile in Egypt. When I was in Palermo, I saw these plants. Their power of desiccation, well known, is enhanced by boiling them after adding glue and fine meal mixed with vinegar. In view of the ingredients of the paper the ancients made, they augmented this power of desiccation to the maximum, for ashing made the medicine even more exsiccatory. Physicians usually ash a medicine, I have found, to enhance the desiccative power, to destroy it, or to eliminate its excessive potency.

We do not have the paper commended by Galen and other ancient authors, so let us see if we have anything to substitute. We do have some kinds of paper made of substances we consider strongly exsiccatory, a property increased if they are burned, and I believe the composition of the papyrus of the ancients was not much different from that of the paper presently available in Sicily. I think that we can use this material in place of papyrus. The ashes steeped in vinegar may be used just as Galen used his burned paper.

In my opinion, our paper is good enough. It is made, as we all know, from pounded linen cloth, softened and reduced to its form with glue. Insofar as the material appertains, we know that linen cloths dry things out and are used by physicians for this purpose in the management of ulcers. Indeed Galen praised Cilician linen cloth (of Lesser Armenia, in Turkey) in treating alopecia, although Cornarius interpreted Galen's word "rakos" to mean wool cloth, which he recommended because, itself exsiccatory, it is appropriate for making exsiccatory medication. If linen dries things out, and if the glue in the paper does so too, and if it is burned in addition, beyond doubt the medicine will be quite exsiccatory. So even if we do not have papyrus, I think our burned paper is satisfactory.

The third point is that the old physicians often used medicines for achor and favus that were called "smegmata" (soapy medicaments). These consisted of abstergent powders that were used for scrubbing and cleansing the body when this was needed. In those days they consisted of saltpeter, burned barley, pumice, broad bean cream, bran, and sulfur. Later ulcers were treated with such medicines, particularly the exudative cases. Another they compounded was from hellabore, alcyon, sulfur, staphisagria, and the test of sepia (cuttlebone).

In using these medicines, it is important to dry the head carefully beforehand, Paullus warned. They are powders, and if applied to a moist skin, their potency would readily be lost. They should, however, sometimes be diluted with a liquid such as oxymel, plain honey, or plain vinegar, as one notes in several of Aetius' essays.

A final point is that both Arabian and Greek physicians almost never used fats in treating such ulcers, but I cannot believe that their reasons were of the best. They must have thought that skin infected with this kind of ulcers becomes hot, and that, since fats themselves are easily burned, fats would enhance the heat of the sores and of the materia. On this account I advise that such fats be avoided insofar as possible, to prevent the reactivation of chronic ulcers.

How can liniments or other medication be kept dry on the head? In my experience the best solution is a felt hat or some kind of cap, tied on with ivy leaves. After dusting the powder on or applying the liniment, the scalp should be protected by the felt covering with a light linen bandage over it. If parts other than the head are affected, ivy leaves can be sewed together and applied in the most convenient way. The ivy itself is moderately exsiccative and repellent and helps to remove the deformed humors.

BOOK ONE, CHAPTER TEN

ON TINEA

THE DRY SORES of the scalp that now follow, as fully described by the Arabs as by the Greeks, are all of them included by Avicenna within the title, "dry sahafati." These are the ulcers that corrupt the scalp and hair. Foul material oozes from them, dry or moist matter of bad odor, and crusting occurs that disfigures the head, even the whole countenance. The sores, recent or old, are in either case usually included in the name "tinea." I say usually because the Arabs and some Latins included moist sores of the scalp within the connotation of "tinea." They are so called from the grub "tinea" that eats away clothing.

Many authors, Nicolaus of Florence among them, have thought that our tinea is the moist sahafati of the Arabs, but they are controverted by the appearance of the disease, for dry sahafati is generated from a melancholic and bilious humor. Indeed both the color and the essential features of our tinea indicate its origin from melancholic and bilious humors, so it is unimaginable that our tinea is not the dry sahafati. The testimony of Avenzoar is confirmatory. He described it under two titles, tinea and moist sahafati. One must conclude that these two diseases are different and not, as Nicolaus thought, the same. Although Avenzoar did not describe our tinea completely, yet moist sahafati does occasionally change into the dry type or into tinea itself.

The immediate cause of this condition, according to Avicenna, is actually the melancholic humor. Mixed with it is an acute, moist quality that obliterates and dries out the powers of expulsion, obliging the body to work against itself and, when excreted, this provokes ulceration.

The mediate and more remote causes are as a whole a complex of six abnormal factors. First of all are bad foods. Contagion is among the causes; if any disease is contracted through contagion, this one is, without a doubt. A hereditary tendency promotes it. Inept treatment of achor and favus may induce contagion, and for this reason we must be on guard as to what course cases of achor and favus take, for bad treatment of them in their early stages will of itself explain why a considerable proportion of the poor are infected with the disease. Sometimes other diseased conditions of the scalp exist, and from them this condition may arise, as Avicenna said.

It may be asked whether the disease was mentioned by the Greeks. I have never been able to find a clear description by any Greek author. However, I think that achor, so named by Alexander from the melancholic humor, refers specifically to our tinea and to the dry sahafati of the Arabs. One can see that the melancholic achor of Alexander plainly does not represent the tinea we are discussing.

Many of the features of these ulcers were described by William the Surgeon. Most important is the appearance of dry scales, sometimes saffron in color, sometimes ashy, occasionally greenish and even black. Little or no humor exudes from them, but the humor itself is full of poison, as if quite venomous. Furthermore, once corrupted, the hairs fall out, and this is a diagnostic feature whereby tinea can be differentiated easily from other diseases. Almost all cases terminate in alopecia and ophiasis. Guido de Cauliaco (Guy de Chauliac), an excellent surgeon, insisted that he had seen this condition terminate in lepra and severe pediculosis.

The literature suggests that there are two kinds of tinea, the one curable, the other not. In the incurable kind the skin appears tough and testaceous (like a shell). Along with corrosion of the hairs, many crusts may be present.

In managing this disease a regimen must be established, a prime necessity, because, if it is disregarded, the generation of defective humors continues. Avicenna warned that sweet things should be avoided particularly, such as dates. He gave these precedence because they were popular among his own people. He objected to all acrid, sharp, salty, coarse, and excessively hot foods. He recommended a diet containing well leavened bread and doves and other small birds, preserved in vinegar. He spoke highly of tasteless dishes. While we note that vinegar is recommended in this condition by many authors, it is to be approved only when mixed with other foods. Alone it is quite harmful and objectionable because, as mentioned by Hippocrates, it promotes the influx of melancholic humor. Haly Abbas gave his patients moist foods and advised nose drops of almond oil, gourd oil, or oil of violets.

After establishing this regimen, one must attend to the elimination of the defective humors, which involve the whole body, the head particularly. They must be prepared first, being otherwise difficult to eliminate. For this purpose a syrup such as the following could be used. Take 1 handful each of leaves of fumaria, asplenium, bryony, and borage. Make a decoction in the usual way. Take 5 ounces of the mixture and add 1 ounce each of syrup of saporrex and syrup of borage juice, and ½ ounce of oxymel. Mix.

When the patient is taking a syrup of this sort, bloodletting must be considered, and one must heed what we have said about the moist ulcers. If indications of blood are present or if the deformed humors are much mixed with blood, then by all means venisection should be performed, and it should be done on the side of the body where the seat of the illness seems to be.

Once prepared, the humors should soon be purged. If the offensive ones are melancholic and bilious, then medicine should be chosen that most effectively draws these out, such as cochia with hellebore pills, hiera of Pacchius with hellebore, and pills of lapis lazuli. If a draught is preferred, I often use the following. Take ½ handful of bryony leaves, 1½ drams each of senna leaves and flowers of thyme, 1 dram of black hellebore bark, and ½ dram each of betony seeds, citrus seeds, and scordium. Soak in whey of goat's milk, let stand overnight, and late in the morning express the mixture. Take 5 ounces of this, 2 scruples of rhubarb troches, 7 grains of violet pastils with scammony, and 2½ drams of dilute syrup of violets. Mix, and give to the patient. This draught, as one recognizes from its composition, effectively purges melancholic and bilious humors. It may be repeated if necessary.

We now turn to the local medication, observing that repellents are never used. Since the materia is dry, the humor is so thick and stubborn that it cannot be eliminated by repellents, and if they are used the humor becomes the more deeply entrenched and, I might say, even worse. Thus we must use medicines that attenuate, exsiccate, consume, and penetrate into the deepest parts.

Before these are presented, however, two points must receive consideration. First, hair, if it is present, must be removed by tweezers or some depilating wax, which shortly I shall discuss. The second point concerns whether the disease is recent and milder or old and more rebellious. In milder cases one uses milder medicines, but in stubborn cases, one must go to the extreme and most active agents.

The way I manage a rather mild case of tinea is as follows. First I order the removal of the infected hairs with tweezers, then the vigorous rubbing of the entire affected area with a powder made of equal parts of cuttlebone and saltpeter. A day or two later I order the washing of the head with the following mixture. Take 1 handful each of bryony roots and white lily roots and 2 handfuls each of mallow, fumaria, and strong sorrel. Boil these in 10 pounds of water until a fourth is consumed. Express the mixture and add 1 cyathus (ounce) of urine. Make a decoction. I wash the head and massage and extract hairs on alternate days. After exsiccation I anoint with oil of sweet almonds, nut oil, or chicken fat. This treatment has failed me seldom in the mild cases of tinea that I was managing.

If the disease is more severe and stubborn, more recalcitrant to treatment, a stronger method must be employed. Modern surgeons are likely to prefer diluted quicksilver to all other medicines. While the Greek writers did not recommend it, nor did Galen know of its wonderful capabilities, yet the Arabs did, Avicenna in particular. There are some who fear the use of mercury, persuaded in their view by reasons that are not bad. It is hazardous, for the affected parts are close to the brain, and there is danger that such a poisonous medicine might reach the brain. Certainly I advise in all diseases of the head that less extreme agents be tried first, but if they are not successful, one may resort to mercury.

In old recalcitrant tinea I usually use a variety of medicines made of lime, copper, vitriol, sulfur, and such things, which are highly successful in the treatment of all tineas and in the elimination of all corruption, but, as I have said, these are given only after the hairs have been removed from the diseased areas. The following is a formula I am in the habit of using. Take 3 ounces each of fumaria juice, scabiosa, borage, strong lapathum, and vinegar. Add 1 pound of old oil. Boil in a double boiler until the liquids and vinegar are consumed, then sprinkle in the following powders. Take ½ dram each of hellebore, sulfur vivum, chalcanthite, orpiment, quicklime, alum and gall, and add 2 drams of copper green. Grind and sift carefully. Then mix with the oil previously formulated, and add pine tar and wax sufficient to make a plaster to cover the whole affected region of the scalp. If the wax plaster is used after the measures we have mentioned have been carried out, and if the disease is not absolutely incurable, we may always hope for optimum success.

Another important and bad feature of this disease is that this disordered skin continually corrupts its own nutrient and regenerates defective humors. Thus one must constantly and energetically remove the defective humors that are produced. Therefore in the younger patients I give cochia pills with hellebore every eighth day, or hiera of Pacchius alone. Quite often I use syrup of polypody with infusion of hellebore.

Heretofore I have said the hair should be removed with tweezers or with a psilother (depilatory unguent). So we need to know the composition of psilothers as given by Galen and others. According to Galen there are three kinds of dissolution of the hair, that which weakens the hairs, that which depilates temporarily, and that which completely destroys them. Things that attenuate the hair and those that extirpate it are never called psilothers, except one that I have found, a white bryony (ampeloleuce), a psilother so called because of its excellence in removing hair.

Agents that remove hair temporarily are called psilothers. They have an erosive and destructive character. Among them are orpiment, realgar, arsenic, and quicklime, all of them corrosive, burning down the hair but not harming the roots.

Many precautions must be considered in using these medicines. First, they must not be given if there is a chance that the skin is too firm, for the harder the skin, the dryer it becomes, but when the skin contains some moisture, they may be used more safely.

Secondly, certain medicines for the removal of hair are never applied alone but always are mixed with something emplastic (glutinous) that will check their fiery, destructive power. Three medicines with these features have been used, I find, according to Galen, quoting Crito: starch, barley water, and rice water (juice of oriza). To make a depilatory, take equal parts of quicklime and orpiment, a sufficient amount of barley water, and a little vinegar. Make a paste watery enough to smear.

Thirdly, one must see to it that these medicines are left on only so long as they do not blister. Because of their heat, they are apt to blister and ought not be left on too long. As soon as they have dissolved the hair, they should be removed with a bath or lotion. If it were asked what the difference is between a dropax and a psilother of this kind, it is true that a dropax will remove the hair. Oribasius, that learned physician, made the distinction that a psilother does less work, leaves the skin soft, and plucks it superficially. A dropax does not work this way, but leaves the texture in better condition and firmer.

After applying a psilother two things may happen. First, the area may smell foul, and secondly, the skin may look rather black. To eliminate the odor, Rhazes recommended rubbing the area with sandalwood, bran, or saffron. Rubbing these on, alone or with other agents, will eliminate the smell the psilother produced. To remove the black discoloration Rhazes recommended a decoction of chick peas or of broad bean meal and chick peas, that I think highly to be recommended.

This portrait reproduced by Simili (1942) was taken from the volume published in Florence in 1856 by the Pietro Conti publishers, "De Arte Gymnastica," 6 Books by H. Mercurialis Translated for the First Time into the Italian Language by the priest, Giovanni Rimaldi of Forli. The engraver is not identified. This information was provided by Dr. Walter Vichi of the Forli Institute of Arts and Culture.

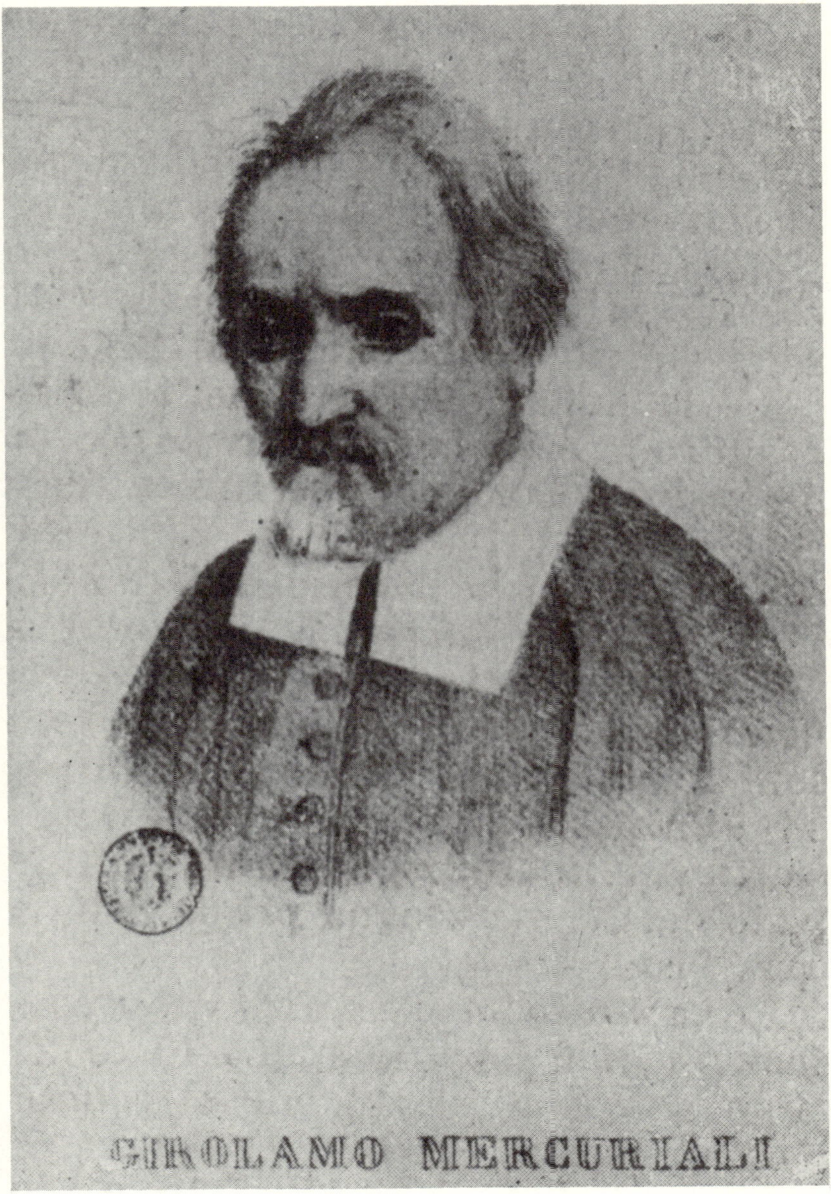

GIROLAMO MERCURIALI

BOOK ONE, CHAPTER ELEVEN

ON PSYDRACHIA, HELCYDRIA, SYCOSIS, AND EXANTHEMATA

IN ADDITION to the diseases of the scalp that we have described heretofore, there are others that are to be found in the last chapter of a book of Galen's. These have been discussed by other Greek writers in various essays and are four or five in number: (1) psydrachia, (2) helcydria, or small ulcers (Gr elkydrion, dim of elkos, wound, sore, L ulcus), (3) sycosis, or "fici" (figs), and (4) exanthemata (eruptions that characterize eruptive fevers). All these were listed by Haly Abbas among the varieties of tinea.

Psydrachia, as Paullus and Alexander gave the definition, are small ulcers of the scalp that resemble those which usually break out on the skin. Cornelius Celsus defined psydrachia somewhat differently, describing the lesions as whitish pustules that are rather firm and pointed, and from which moist matter can be expressed. Julius Pollux differs from others in defining the affection as a fiery efflorescence of the scalp that undergoes spontaneous ulceration. All agree that a psydrachion is a small ulcer.

Exanthemata, on the other hand, are simply the eruptions that appear on the scalp exactly like the rashes that involve the whole body.

Helcydria, so-called, as we learn from Aetius, are small, firm, red sores in the scalp of the shape of little nipples, from which a thin bloody ichor exudes. Celsus was apparently speaking about all these small ulcers when he wrote that, dry or moist, they develop from pustules and are accompanied by pruritus as well as inflammation and pain, and material, purulent, sanguineous, or both, exudes from them.

All of these scalp conditions seem to have about the same cause, which is undoubtedly a great ebullition of blood and phlegm in the head itself. For this reason Galen rightly concluded that the methods of treatment are the same for all. Because the diseases involve children most frequently, no author has mentioned venisection. A dietary regimen is of primary importance, and it should be required of both the child and the nurses, and they must avoid the things that promote accumulation of defective humors. Galen recommended also purgation of the head and body, and he thought highly of his own aloes pills, which we shall examine a little later.

After purgation of the body, he instructed us to take up the local remedies, which, I find, are of two types, the one gentle and handed down from Galen, the other more vigorous that was proposed by Paullus and Alexander.

Galen's remedies were melilot and fenugreek, powdered and steeped in vinegar, to be rubbed onto the scalp and the diseased areas. Likewise effective are bitter almonds. When ground fine and chewed, these are quite abstergent and exsiccative. When chewed, they acquire something from the saliva of a softening and dissipative quality. As Avicenna said, in speaking of the kinds of humors, wheat when chewed is softened and swollen by the saliva, and this is likewise true of bitter almonds because the small fragments are well mixed together. Raw lily root soaked in vinegar is fairly effective.

"Bulbs," too, were recommended. One notes that these were used by the ancients as medicine but also more commonly as food, but no record is left for us to know what kind of bulbs they really were. As a substitute for them, I usually use a bulb known as ascalonium (shallot). This agent, with which I am familiar in treating this kind of disease, is a mild one.

Here is another topical remedy. Take 2 drams of incense and 1 dram each of powdered pomegranate rind, saltpeter, and bran. Pulverize, soak in vinegar, and rub on the head. The strength of this preparation lies between the gentler and the more vigorous.

The most vigorous are those made of silver spume, blue vitriol, and lye, all of which were discussed by Paullus and Alexander.

Celsus recommended two measures as especially useful in curing these cases. First, he required that the patients walk and exercise a good deal and, if they cannot, they should be carried. Secondly, the patients should reduce the intake of food and avoid irritating and wearing affairs.

Certain conditions of the scalp are called "the scab" (scabious diseases, L scabiosa), and Avenzoar discussed them especially fully, but do not be deceived, for this weighty author actually included all kinds of achors and favi within the title. Some have called achors and favi "sagrus," which is what Avenzoar called the scabious ones, the achors and favi of the scalp. In this condition the skin comes off so that the whole head looks as if flayed.

In such excoriated cases, the best treatment is olive leaves steeped in rose honey and applied as a poultice, an almost painless treatment that brings about replacement of the skin quickly.

With regard to "fici," (figs, i.e. kerions), or "fications," of the scalp, Oribasius and Paullus described these lesions as round, rather firm, and reddish, sometimes painful. Mostly they involve the head but may occur on other parts of the body. Haly Abbas in enumerating the varieties of tinea said that there are two kinds, of which one is hard and rounded on the surface and the other contains a rather heavy material resembling figs, which explains the names. Cornelius Celsus described the condition more clearly, noting that a certain sore called "sykosis" in Greek is so called because of the resemblance to a fig (Gr sykon) in which the meat is excrescent. But this feature is common to all, so Celsus put the two species together, the one characterized by hard, round sores, the other, by moist sores of various shapes. A small amount of sticky liquid exudes from the hard type. From the moist type come a greater quantity of humor and an evil smell. Both develop on the hairy scalp, but they may occur in the beard, where they are firm, solid, and sticky. The moist type involves particularly the hairy regions. While Celsus' description seems somewhat different from those of Paullus, Oribasius, and Haly Abbas, one can see that they are practically identical.

As to the treatment of "fici," I find Cornelius Celsus and the Greeks differed. Celsus praised elaterium, finely ground flaxseed boiled in water, or figs cooked in water, or tetrapharmicon plaster dissolved in vinegar, and Eretrian earth, all of them quite bland.

Paullus and the Greeks apparently recommended stronger things, advising the use of alum, blue vitriol, scales of bronze, lye, and other medicines that certainly seem stronger. The discrepancy is due, I believe, simply to the fact that Cornelius Celsus always used milder medication, while the Greeks used more daring remedies.

Earlier I stated that Galen recommended his aloes pills for purging the humors in the treatment of these conditions, so we should now like to know their composition, what value they may possess, and how to compound them correctly. He described the composition as follows. Take 2 drams each of aloes and scammony, 1 dram of colocynth, and 1 dram of wormwood juice. Mix carefully and make a catapotion. Galen's intent with these pills was simply to purge the body of bile especially and of phlegm secondarily, so he included two ingredients for purging bile, aloes and scammony. We have learned from Mesue that aloes purges bile, so he thought its use unnecessary in winter when bile is not a dominant humor. Galen actually disapproved the use of aloes in old people, who do not have much bile. It is clear that colocynth eliminates phlegm. So Galen's purpose, to remove bile first and phlegm later, was evident.

With regard to the composition, two matters deserve review as to why Galen said he did not wish to incorporate gum mastic and bdellium, as Serenus Quintus habitually did. Galen rejected these, he wrote, and promised to give the reason elsewhere. There is reasonable doubt that the medicines were properly corrected. Since there are 2 drams of scammony and 1 dram of colocynth, one sees nothing to correct the vigor and potency of the medication. In my opinion, and rightly so I believe, Galen must have thought the mastic and bdellium antagonistic, so that the medicine was corrected as it stood. Undoubtedly with the potency of its ingredients it would remove bile even from regions as remote as the head, after the stimulated bilious humors had been loosened. Thus bdellium and gum mastic, themselves sluggish and gentle, would reduce the harshness and excessive strength of the other ingredients, and I think Galen was right in omitting them.

That this medicine is not lacking in corrective power we may easily understand from Mesue's chapter on aloes, where he described it as having the greatest virtue of all. Almost all other purges weaken the stomach and the main viscera, while aloes, he said, will correct and ameliorate the defects of other medicines. From these quotations we may be quite satisfied that aloes is the best as a corrective of other medications.

This being so, two important points stand out clearly regarding the composition of these pills. First, the viscera and stomach must be protected from the ill effects of scammony and colocynth. Aloes, with its thickness, blunts their harshness little by little. Secondly, while it corrects, nevertheless it does not eliminate the purgative features of the other medicines, but actually enhances them. Since of itself it purges bile, it is actually an adjuvant to their qualities.

One understands then why the ancients, especially the Arabs, always put aloes in the formula of practically all pills containing strong medication, and we understand why Galen omitted bdellium and gum mastic in formulating his pills even though Serenus Quintus included them.

One may ask why Galen included wormwood juice in treating alopecia and ophiasis, while for small ulcers of the scalp he wished to include the juice of brassica (cabbage) and not wormwood. I reply that since these juices are included merely to formulate and compound the medicine, it does not matter much which we choose. If there is any reason, however, for including them, I think it is because brassica juice is somewhat antagonistic to ulcers, pustules, and tumors, and that is why Galen selected it. In the treatment of alopecia and ophiasis, he made use of wormwood juice, supposedly helpful to the stomach and liver both, because these diseases are due to a deformity of the humors and because both arise from defects of the stomach and liver. But perhaps, as I have said, Galen chose one juice or the other for no reason at all.

It may be asked what we know of the quantity of the medicine. Galen gave us a measure when he said a catapotion of eleven pills, each of chick-pea size, should be taken one at a time. It is not easy to find the weight of a chick-pea-size pill, but one lupine, I find, weighs a third of a scruple, and a chick-pea does not differ much from a lupine. Some grains of the one weigh the same as some of the other. So I think the weight of a chick-pea is about the same as that of lupine. If we calculate the dose at eleven thirds of a scruple, it comes to about four scruples. One must keep the constitution and condition of the patient in mind, because for the most part children and adolescents cannot stand that much, so we might reduce the dose but would never increase it.

And so this essay on diseases of the scalp is ended.

HIERONYMUS MERCURIALIS ON DISEASES OF THE SKIN

SECOND BOOK ON DISEASES OF THE SKIN OF THE WHOLE BODY

BOOK TWO, CHAPTER ONE

CLASSIFICATION

FOLLOWING the discussion of disorders of the scalp, we come to the consideration of those of the whole body, not in the sense that the entirety of the skin is diseased but rather in the sense that the disease may involve any part of the skin. Many diseases that occur in the skin originate elsewhere, and I will not discuss these but will limit myself to diseases that seem to originate in the skin itself or only a little deeper.

Disorders of this kind seem to me to fall into two classes based on the color and on the roughness and smoothness of the skin. I shall discuss the ones involving color first. Some of these are of internal origin, such as jaundice, but I shall not discuss either black or yellow jaundice, for they require an independent essay.

With regard to color, there are two diseases, "leuce" and "alphos" (see chapter following).

With regard to roughness and smoothness, there are four: impetigo or lichen, pruritus, scabies or psora, and lepra. I do not propose to discuss at this time some other diseases that can alter the roughness and smoothness of the skin, such as tumors and apostemes (abscesses).

BOOK TWO, CHAPTER TWO

ON LEUCE AND ALPHOS

BEFORE beginning to discuss the defects of skin color, I must describe the natural color. Although it seems that no rule can be given as to the color, nevertheless there are two features to be observed in almost all individuals, or at least in the majority of them. First, the color is a mixture of white and red, thus, indeed, Galen wrote that the skin is, as it were, a fibrillar structure (nervum) suffused with blood, his words plainly suggesting that the natural color of the skin is a mixture of red and white. Secondly, the color is not the same in all parts of the body but is diverse. The cheeks are of one color, the hands another, the feet yet another, and this is true of each part of the body. Thus the color will either remain normal in all parts of the body or will be altered, a little pale or a little more livid, in which case an abnormality in the color exists.

Such abnormalities have two names, according to the Greeks, "leuce" and "alphos," and the latter may be either white (albus) or black (niger). The Latins called these abnormalities by the same name, "vitiligo," a word derived from either "vitium" (blemish) or "vitulum" (small blemish), as Festus said. Cornelius Celsus included alphos and leuce within the title, "vitiligo." The Arabs, using other names, called leuce "albara," with white and black varieties, and called alphos "morphea," likewise with white and black varieties. Thus the Greeks used only one name, leuce, and the Arabs had two varieties of leuce, the white and the black.

Cornelius Celsus differed from both the Greeks and Arabs, for he called white alphos simply alphos and called black alphos "melana." He classed all of these conditions, as I have said, within the title "vitiligo," some cases of which he called alphos and others leuce, as the Greeks did.

Leuce, as Galen wrote, and also Aetius, comes from the word for white, and Galen said explicitly that leuce is white like poplar. As whiteness appears in the tree in the form of down, so it appears in the skin in this condition. Paullus of Aegina and Aelius Promotus in their medical texts said that leuce is simply the change of the skin color to white that is brought about by viscid and dense phlegm. Galen said it is one of the diseases brought about through changes of the solid parts. Indeed he said that the flesh, too, is changed in this disease.

Disease of this kind occurs apparently because of an error in the nutritive faculty when this faculty produces phlegm, or at any rate pituitous (mucous) blood, instead of blood. When nourished by this for a long time, the flesh develops a condition peculiar in that it readily converts everything into this whiteness, as a result of which it is no longer normal flesh but may be said to be whitened flesh. Yet even if badly nourished, it still remains flesh, but it is so transformed that it will be of a white color instead of ruddy. Similarly, Galen said, we see shellfish and oysters become white.

If the flesh in leuce becomes white in this way, one may ask why the hands are attacked by the disease rather than the feet. For in leuce we do see the hands more frequently involved. Alexander solved the problem when he explained why the feet suffer less than the hands. The feet are subject to more exercise, so the phlegmatic humor in them is to a greater degree removed, and this explains why their flesh is not attacked, whereas the hands, which are not so active, do not consume the phlegm and therefore suffer more from leuce than the feet.

These considerations make it easy to understand that the material cause of the disease is actually none other than viscid and thick phlegm. The divine Plato wrote that white phlegm has two effects in the body. If it is retained in the brain, he said, it will cause epilepsy, and if it is retained outside the brain and begins to vent through the exterior of the body, it will cause alphos and vitiligo. Plato was aware, then, that leuce and alphos come from white phlegm, although Ficinus did not phrase this passage sufficiently clearly. The efficient cause of this disease is none other than the weakness of the nutritive power. This, then, is the nature of the disease called leuce by the Greeks and albara by the Arabs, and these are its causes.

Alphos, which the Arabs included within the name "morphea," has almost the same origin as leuce except that the lesions may be black because of a black humor. But alphos and leuce are different. The lesions in alphos are white, I say, first because they alter the color of the skin, and also they are called alphos appropriately, according to Aetius, because of the whitening, "ato ton alphainein," a phrase which to the ancients implied that in alphos a change occurred. Both species of alphos, white as well as black, differ from leuce in that the latter alters the skin to a greater extent, so that the hairs, too, undergo the change. Furthermore we have the testimony of Aristotle, who said that only man is subject to leuce because he has a more tender skin and only man becomes white haired. Alphos affects only the surface of the skin and does not alter the hairs, but in a more advanced stage, it usually does change the hairs and progresses deeper insidiously.

The Latin physician, Celsus, no less assiduous than eloquent, propounded a number of distinguishing features for differentiating alphos from leuce. First, he said, both disorders evolve insidiously, in some cases quickly, in others slowly. He felt that the lesions in alphos are white without significant roughness, and that, while they might be a little rough, they are not consistently so. In some cases of alphos the white macules spread throughout the skin, but the lesions in leuce have continuity; yet, while those in alphos are sometimes rather broad, the main difference is that in leuce continuity is apparent, but never in alphos.

Black alphos differs in no way from white except in color. Just as white alphos consists of individual white guttae (drop-like spots), so black alphos consists of individual black guttae. Celsus added, too, that alphos is not especially difficult to cure. It is to be noted that Celsus said "not very difficult," while Pollux thought it "dysiatos," hard to cure. Leuce is never, or rarely ever, curable. Once contracted, it just does not go away. Nor do the words of Aetius leave any doubt, for he wrote that in alphos there might appear to be scales, as it were, not true squamae but, as Celsus said, guttae that simulate scales.

Avicenna made a distinction between the materiae of leuce and alphos when he described that of leuce as thicker and that of alphos as more subtle. It may be asked why the Greeks did not recognize two kinds of leuce, as the Arabs did. I reply that the Greeks were right, for they derived the name from the word for whiteness. To speak of "black leuce" is as unthinkable as to speak of "black whiteness." The Arabs, however, using the name "albara," could properly distinguish two kinds. But the fact must not be ignored that black albara, according to Avicenna and the Arabs, was not a kind of vitiligo, and not a disease involving the color of the skin. It was a variety of excoriating impetigo, actually the "lepra Graecorum."

Here one should not overlook the fact that there is a difference between leuce and leucophlegmasia, the latter being, as Galen taught, a kind of dropsy, a condition, sometimes called anasarca by the Greeks, in which almost all the blood becomes phlegmatic and fills the entirety of the body. There is another kind of leucophlegmasia that Galen described as a disease in which the flesh becomes soft, somewhat swollen, and white. It is apparent that this is not leuce, a disease in which the flesh is not swollen but, rather, is flat or depressed.

The antecedent causes of leuce and alphos are many. First, as Hippocrates said, is the time of year when vitiligo and leuce actually develop. This is because the bodily humors, activated by the warmth of the air, flow naturally to the exterior parts and, once embedded in the skin, create after awhile not only vitiligo but also leuce. The geographic region, too, seems to be an antecedent cause. Plutarch said that foreigners and Jews are especially susceptible to leuce. We have in fact a letter of Aeschines reporting that among the Delians he saw white vitiligo in nearly all of them. Seneca added that certain waters may convey not only scabies but also vitiligo and an ugly variety of "whiteness," either on wetting the skin or on ingestion, and that the dew has this injurious property. An ugly variety of "whiteness," it is to be noted, is an erroneous interpretation, a false reading of the text, which ought to read of "alphos." This reading would plainly make sense.

Sex and age likewise contribute to the production of the disease. It is handed down to us from Aristotle that children and women suffer from leuce less than men, but it is worse in older women. He added exhaled vapors (spiritus exitus) as a cause. Children do not contract the disease because their bodies are denser and do not have this exhalation, and also women are seldom affected because their bodies are relieved and made firm through the cleansing effect of menstruation, while the bodies of old women are of a flabbier construction and, like old buildings, are more subject to cracks (hiantia).

Avenzoar wrote that white morphea comes from excessive and frequent exercise and black morphea from not rubbing down after the bath. The misuse of cupping glasses often causes the condition, as we learn from Avicenna. As the cup draws blood to the skin, it draws phlegm too, and this when retained in the skin is likely to make alphos and leuce by its viscosity. Debility is another cause. The spleen is one of the factors productive of black alphos, as explained by Galen. When the stomach cannot eliminate the melancholic humor from the circulation (ambitu) in the body, that which is retained makes this kind of disorder.

The body habitus is of itself an antecedent cause of leuce and alphos. Rhazes said he had seen individuals with small muscles and wide veins involved with this disease, a fact confirmed by Galen himself. There are certain deadly diseases that produce these conditions. The wasting sickness (tabes) is one to which Hippocrates referred.

I may be asked whether the condition may be due to contagion, which apparently may cause nearly any skin condition. Alexander wrote that vitiligo is by no means contagious, and he offered in explanation the fact that, since the phlegm which causes the disease is viscid and thick, it cannot easily be communicated from one skin to another. A further reason may be added. Since this disease results from a cold and viscid humor from which no evaporation comes, there can be no contagious exhalation, and this disease cannot possibly be communicated by way of vapors. Thus it is clear that this disease, of all skin diseases, cannot be transmitted by contagion. Avicenna wrote, however, that white vitiligo is sometimes hereditary.

The diagnostic features of black alphos are clear enough. The distinct macules are quite dark, without roughness, excoriation, tenderness, or abnormal warmth. The features differentiating white alphos and leuce are not clear, for characteristic differences are wanting. In leuce, as has been said, there are certainly white spots, but they are continuous so as to be confluent and interconnected in almost all locations. Besides, the hairs are also white. In white alphos the spots are white but separate from one another, and the hairs are not white. This is because the condition does not involve the inner skin as leuce does. Avicenna added another distinguishing characteristic, found in the Greek descriptions. In alphos if the skin is rubbed, blood will come out, but in leuce it is not blood that comes but rather a white materia. Moreover, he said, in leuce the flesh is not sunken where it is not involved, but in the macules the flesh appears somewhat depressed and hollowed.

One can readily see that the disease of the Delians that Aeschines described in his Greek letters, is not true vitiligo, as we have fully annotated heretofore. Even if these people do have white spots on the face and white hair, as he said, still they have swollen necks and breasts (pectora), too, and they perceive some pain, and it is clear that this is not white alphos or vitiligo but is a species of leuce, which we described in accordance with Galen. Finally, all kinds of vitiligo have in common the characteristic, stressed by Lucilius and quoted by Festus, of being disgusting (foeda) but not injurious (odiosa).

As to the prognosis, first, as Cornelius Celsus said, this disease is not of itself dangerous but is only objectionable in appearance and comes from a bad condition of the body. The views of other Greek authorities seem contrary to his. Paullus said that if the top of the skin is punctured in a case of leuce, and blood does not ooze out but rather a white humor, then the disease is incurable and hopeless, so the disease is not without its dangers. Aetius, too, wrote that if the hairy parts become bald in the course of leuce, the case is incurable. Likewise Serapion and Avicenna, following Paullus, said that if leuce involves a large area and enlarges steadily, it is either incurable or very difficult to cure.

Thus there seems to be a contradiction between Celsus and the Greek writers. Yet correctly examined, a difference does not exist. Cornelius Celsus spoke of danger to life in a way suggesting that he meant the disease does not cause death. The Greeks did not say that these conditions are fatal but that they are protracted and so difficult to recover from that the patient hardly ever recovers his health. Some authors, like Appuleius, adducing the authority of Plato, have said that those who suffer from leuce or alphos do not contract epilepsy, but it is far from the truth that Plato said this.

Two questions are to be disposed of before we consider the treatment. The first is whether vitiligo, coming as it does from a phlegmatic humor, can be produced by bile and blood. I raise this question because Nicolaus of Florence was of the opinion that it can. What he said is not in the records of any other physician simply because the disease so rarely comes from any humor other than phlegm.

The second question is whether vitiligo and alphos are true diseases or only symptoms. That they are diseases Galen seems clearly to have stated, when he assigned vitiligo and alphos a place among the diseases due to changes in the solid parts. This seems to have been the opinion of Plato, where he wrote that if phlegm secures a passageway (spiramen, a breathing hole) to the exterior, it tints the body with various colors and produces vitiligo. He seemed to consider other diseases to be of this kind, as if he clearly meant that they are diseases. Nor should the opinion of Plato on this subject be disregarded, for Galen in citing it said that Hippocrates concurred. On the other hand, there is a citation where Galen listed vitiligo among the symptoms that represent altered qualities, that is, alterations of colors. The explanation is, in part, that diseases of this sort primarily and of themselves do not harm the operations of the body, so they should in no wise be called "diseases."

As for the solution of the first question, it is to be said that neither vitiligo nor alphos can come from blood or yellow bile. They certainly cannot be produced from blood because, as we have learned from Galen, diseases of this kind occur because of a defect of the alterative faculty. Where the blood is best in the body and carries back neither bile nor phlegm, and is pure, none of this defect of the alterative faculty will appear. So we cannot say that it is made of blood. But it may be said that blood can be diffused widely throughout the surface of the skin and become attached to the body as sanguineous macules, either discrete or continuous. I reply that this might occur, although such a condition should not be called either vitiligo or alphos, the essential character of which is that the alterative faculty is defective, as Galen and Avicenna noted.

That vitiligo cannot come from bile is easy to prove. According to Galen's views, vitiligo and alphos are due to coldness. To the extent that bile is abundant, coldness is absent and heat is dominant. Furthermore, if bile changes the color of the skin, it will cause either erysipelas, pruritus, or some ulcerative affliction. Thus origination from bile cannot explain the development or spreading of vitiligo.

With regard to the second question, one must reply that, as Galen taught, these conditions are symptoms, not true diseases because change of color never of itself harms the operations of the body. Although some have thought that tactile sensibility (sensum tactus) is impaired in this condition, I say that it is not damaged or, if damaged at all, the change of color is not the cause but rather a distemper of coldness, which is as it were the disease itself to which this symptom is attributable. The fact that a cold distemper is present is confirmed by the long discourse Galen gave where he showed, in accordance with the views of Aristotle, that the body parts when so nourished are changed with respect to color by the nutriment. Taking leuce as an example, he said that this disease is due to the frequent influx of phlegmatic materia into the flesh. Thus the flesh is changed by an alteration effected by phlegm and as a consequence is made colder than normal. If the flesh is so changed, then one must agree that the alterative faculty itself is changed. Undoubtedly the alteration comes about through the action of native heat, by the alteration and diminution of which the alterative faculty is necessarily diminished.

It may be asked how the alterative faculty is vitiated in this condition. Galen wrote that in vitiligo and alphos the assimilative faculty is altered, but even if it is damaged, the alterative faculty is not, necessarily. I reply that both the assimilative and àlterative faculties are damaged, because even if the liver produces, distributes, and supplies good blood, nevertheless this cannot be assimilated, because the alterative faculty performs the operation of assimilation, and, since it has been damaged, the assimilative faculty is damaged too. Hence there is no contradiction in the words of Galen, because the assimilative faculty is not vitiated unless the alterative faculty is as well.

With regard to black alphos, the question arises as to how it comes about and whether it comes from a hot, burning distemper or a dry, cold one. I think it comes from a cold one, for two reasons. First, all authors say that the origins of black alphos and of leuce are the same. Secondly, black alphos comes by the nature of things from a melancholia spread throughout skin that is cold and dry, as has been satisfactorily established.

To continue, I reply that our authorities, Galen and Plato, when they called vitiligo and alphos diseases, used the name "disease" for both. So the name, diseases, applies to all of these abnormalities, not entirely appropriately, but to the extent that they actually harm the operations of the body. For the same reason, Galen called ophiasis and alopecia diseases.

In treatment there are two principles, although treatment is the same for both white alphos and leuce. In the first place, the cold distemper of the exterior of the body must be removed. Secondly, the particular symptom, the alteration of the color, must be eliminated. Since this symptom stems from the disease, clearly from a distemper, such effort is requisite for its destruction, because it is fomented by the humors themselves. These are to be drawn from the body first. It is not sufficient to rid the body of the phlegmatic humors that are present unless new ones are kept from developing. Therefore a regimen must be established that will prohibit the development of phlegmatic humors.

It may be asked whether there need be much concern as to the regimen and the evacuations. The Greeks seem not to have mentioned these matters. I say that concern is necessary and that the Greeks did not mention it because they assumed it would be attended to. Moreover, it is an invariable and standard medical precept that strong local medicines, whatever kinds may be used for treating vitiligo, are never to be administered unless the correct regimen has already been established and the whole body purged. On this account the Arabs, who were more painstaking than the Greeks regarding their methods of treatment, did mention the diet and purgation and gave copious instructions as to these necessary measures.

First, the air should be warm and dry, and if this is not to be had naturally, it should be obtained artificially. It is easy to see that such air is helpful in this condition, for those who live in the warm, eastern regions do not get vitiligo.

Sleeping and wakefulness should be regulated, and one should sleep rather than merely rest lying awake, for, as Galen wrote, nothing is quite like sleep for digesting the undigested juices. Since there is an abundance of undigested juices in these diseases, one must get enough sleep.

All activities and exercises done at the right time are wonderfully helpful in these diseases, for they put warmth into the members, both external and internal. By this heat, the cold constitution is after a time readily disposed of, and a warmer one takes its place. Depression and grief should be avoided, and sexual activity, too, is disapproved, although Rhazes would not prohibit it completely, particularly if done on an empty stomach, and Avicenna concurred. Nevertheless, it is important to abstain even if only rarely does it weaken the native heat and make the body parts colder.

Sometimes vomiting after a meal is a useful measure, as Serapion noted, for by this means the humors are evacuated which, undigested in the stomach, reach the liver through the mesenteric veins, humors that control the constitution and not only make these diseases worse but also usually promote new ones.

One must be greatly concerned with food and drink. Aristotle taught that the colors of animals are easily changed by changes of food and especially of drink, a fact confirmed by Galen. It is said that if cattle drink certain waters, their hair may become red, sometimes black, sometimes white.

In these diseases the drinking of water is usually useless, even harmful. Paullus and Avicenna recommended on the contrary drinking old, strong, good wine. Cold and moist foods should all be avoided, such as fish and smelly vegetables, especially cold foods, grain, meal, and, finally, all the things that tend to create cold, phlegmatic juices. Paullus prohibited all oils because, I think, they usually make the body more moist, for he added that foods should be taken dry. Thus Avenzoar rightly highly recommended the meat of doves, exsiccative, and of birds from the mountains, small roasted chickens, partridges, and meats that exsiccate and promote healthy, normal juices. Rhazes warned against sweets and sour foods. Susceptible people should above all avoid pork, on which subject Plutarch is often quoted as having said that foreigners and Jews abstain from it because they are susceptible to the disease and fear it greatly. This is because swine are usually infected with it.

After the dietary regimen has been established, the offensive humors in this disease must be carefully prepared. Those that are cold and thick should be prepared with cutting (incidentibus), heating, and abstergent drugs, such as Byzantine syrup, rose flavored honey, syrup of two roots, syrup of five roots, simple and composite oxymel, and syrup of betony; and from these, along with suitable decoctions, the syrups can be made for preparing these humors.

After the humors have been prepared, they should be eliminated by the drugs that remove the phlegmatic humors especially, among which the best are those compounded of agaric, turpeth, and hiera of colocynth. Here the drugs that best promote urination are to be recommended, too.

Rhazes noted—and it was wise of him—that in this illness purgative medicines are not actually necessary because the materia of this disease is in the superfices of the skin, from which they are difficult to remove with drugs. There are no medicines capable of drawing from the belly and expelling humors that are actually confined in the skin.

It seems ridiculous to me that not a few physicians, on seeing humors in the surface of the skin, are fearful that when drugs are given the humors will be drawn inwardly, but I think this is why the Greek authors omitted mentioning purgative drugs in the treatment of this disease. Avicenna correctly therefore taught that no medicines need be taken unless the abnormal humors lie hidden in the deep recesses of the body. He knew too that medication is unnecessary unless the humors are in the interior.

After purgation we come to the local remedies that are to be applied to the skin itself. On this matter, as Paullus of Aegina taught, there have been various opinions. Some have proposed to burn the skin with fire; others were of the opinion that cauterization should be done with caustics rather than fire. Some, fearing both fire and caustics, thought that the skin should be stained with pigments and dyes. The more potent medicines, in case the job is to be done with medication, are those that are abstergent, divisive (dissecting), and dissolvent. Hippocrates seems to have recommended limewater, which was the practice of the ancients, who were all somewhat bolder in the medication they chose than those who came after them.

For leuce and alphos the medicines ought to be abstergent, penetrating, and dissolving, with this difference, that they need to be more penetrant in leuce than in white alphos because in leuce the humors lie more deeply. There are, however, medicines that are appropriate for the several kinds. Some are strongly abstergent but not strongly dissolvent, such as staphisagria, lupine, spuma maris, caper root, and dry fig leaves. In this category Galen recommended bitter almonds steeped in vinegar. There are other medicines that are strongly dissolvent, both kinds of hellebore, nigella, preserves (condisi), sulfur, laurel, pyrethrum, pepper, castor (beaver musk), the root of the common cucumber, onion, and narcissus bulbs. Oribasius recommended the dung of starlings that have been fed nothing but rice.

These are the kinds of medicines that best dissolve and thin the materia. There are others effective not only as dissolvents but also attrahent, drawing blood to the skin. Of this kind of medicines, called dropaces, are saltpeter, aphroniter (efflorescence or flowers of saltpeter), adarce, species of alcyon, and orpiment. Cornelius Celsus spoke highly of sulfur, frankincense, and lentils steeped in vinegar. Rhazes recommended solatium silvestre.

All these are to be applied according to the indications. First, the abstergent ones alone should be tried and then, if they are not effective, the stronger dissolvent and dissective ones. If the disease does not yield to these, one must resort finally to those which are actively dissolvent and attrahent to the blood, all of which are applied either as plasters or powders to be rubbed on.

Regarding the application of these medicines, three requirements must be observed. First, before any remedy is applied, one must ascertain whether the condition is curable. This is done by a trial of perforation. When the affected area is pricked with a needle, if the humor that emanates is milky, this is no case for medicines because it is incurable. If blood comes out, the case will respond to medicines and should do well on suitable treatment. In this case, the first and best thing to do is to rub the affected part well with a harsh cloth or dry fig leaves, or it may be scarified in several places so as to provide better entry for the medicines so they may act more effectually. Avicenna recommended putting them on during the daytime, for they seem to be more active and penetrant then.

The second point to be observed is that after one has tried all other kinds of medicines, one should not hesitate to try the ones that are rubefacient and vesicating. They are often beneficial when others are not. The outstanding agents for rubefaction and vesication are anacard (cashew), thapsia, cantharides, arsenic, milk of figs, mustard, euphorbia, milk of tithymal, quicklime, and blue vitriol.

If these do not succeed, there is nothing left to do except to use fire itself (the actual cautery). As to its application, Nicolaus of Florence, an illustrious physician, recommended that the burning should be done on the particular parts involved. In support of this view, he adduced the testimony of Paullus, who, he intimated, had said that many cases had been cured this way. I do not like it because it produces ugly scars. To make such scars for removing merely an ugly color does not seem to me a cure but rather a descent from a bad condition to a worse. This was not Paullus' recommendation. The Latin interpreters translated badly: Paullus said only that some have recommended burning. Even I have recommended cauterizing a lesion, but with such moderation as to avoid any danger of objectionable scarring.

Thirdly, one must heed the precept handed down from Avenzoar that whenever local medicines are applied, things must be done to strengthen and fatten the liver. Here all the medicines that can fatten, adjust, and strengthen the liver should be used, both internally and externally. Avenzoar recommended several, to which one may refer in his writings. We have Haly Abbas' diarrhodon confection (diarrhodon Abbatis), outstanding for settling and strengthening the intestines.

Black alphos, although treated in much the same way as white alphos and leuce, has nevertheless certain peculiarities, the principal one being the diet, which, it seemed to Avicenna and the other Arabs, should promote moistening. Thus baths of plain water are to be strongly recommended, also foods that moisten the body, and wine, light or much diluted with water. Avenzoar recommended doves, chicken, and kid's meat. One should refrain from all oils but that of sweet almonds.

As to evacuations in this disease, the Arabic physicians had much to say. Since the materia is for the most part internal, it is expelled better by evacuants. Avicenna was of the opinion that in treating black alphos one should begin with venesection, because this disease is due to the melancholic humor, and the humors that cause disease are usually mixed with the blood. So I judge that if there are any indications of the presence of blood, one should start treatment with bloodletting. Next the humors should be prepared with medication suited to this purpose, such as syrup of lupine, borage juice, and fumitory, apple syrup, and syrup of saporrex. Syrups may be made up of suitable decoctions of these.

The humors thus prepared should be evacuated by medicines with the power of drawing out melancholic humors. The foremost of these apparently are thyme, polypody, black myrobalan, pills of lapis lazuli, black hellebore, hiera of Rufus, and hiera Logodionis.

After evacuation, two things must be done. First the spleen is to be strengthened, for this disease indeed rarely occurs without weakness of it. Secondly, after the spleen has been strengthened, one turns immediately to local medication. As has been said elsewhere, abstergent medication should be tried first. Secondly, desiccative and dissolvent medication should be given, and thirdly, attrahents that draw the blood, and finally the vesicants. Medicines of this kind include the gums, wild rue, mustard, milk of tithymal, and all those we have listed heretofore as rubefacient and vesicant.

As to their use, further consideration should be kept in mind.

First, there are two methods for applying vesicants in this condition. One is to keep it on the affected part until the skin is inflamed and comes away. After the skin has peeled, it is let alone until little by little the areas appear to have been renewed, then one should apply the vesicant again, repeating this many times. The other method is to keep the vesicant on until it brings on a kind of mordication (gnawing sensation), and, as soon as this occurs, it is removed and the skin let alone until this stops. The blister is reapplied, left on only until the gnawing recurs, then removed, and this is done repeatedly.

I have always thought this latter method better, for two reasons. First, blood is drawn gently to the affected part so there is no danger of making an ugly scar, which is the hazard of the former method, which sometimes takes the skin off and leaves a scar. The second point to be kept in mind is that the area should always be soaked with milk after the use of vesicants, for if any trace of unnatural heat from medication remains, milk removes it.

BOOK TWO, CHAPTER THREE

ON PRURITUS

FOLLOWING upon disorders of skin color are those involving the smooth skin, which I have promised to discuss. The ones with which we are here concerned are four in number: pruritus, scabies, or psora, lepra, and the lichens, or impetigines, all accompanied by pruritus.

As Avenzoar clearly noted, the difference between a medicament that induces itching and one that blisters is that the former penetrates deeply, but the latter seems to damage only the surface of the skin. While the affections enumerated apparently are accompanied by itching, this particular essay of ours will be concerned with pruritus because it seems to develop before the others and to degenerate into them very quickly.

By Greek physicians this disease was called "knismos" (itching, tingling, irritation, fretting). In two places Hippocrates called it xysmon (fr Gr xysma, something scraped, planed, filed off), where he spoke of a certain Athenian suffering from pruritus who was cured by means of baths but later died. Erotianus noted in his book that the name "xysmon" was used only by Hippocrates.

Pruritus occurs in two forms, the one mild and relieved simply by scratching, the other more serious, requiring remedies other than scratching. We shall not discuss the former, for it is not difficult to cure—in fact, quite easy—but will discourse on the more serious pruritus.

It is necessary first to note that all the conditions with which pruritus is associated differ from pruritus, for in the other diseases swelling, ulcerations, or excoriations are visible, while in pruritus none of these is present. The flesh appears little altered, harsher in some ways but without noticeable swelling, ulceration, or excoriation. In other conditions associated with pruritus, furthermore, some kind of excretion emanates from the skin. In pruritus nothing comes from the skin except, as Avicenna said, some furfuraceous flakes, and not even these unless the skin is torn by the nails.

Some authorities have defined pruritus as an abnormal sensation that leads to scratching induced at a particular place from a continued dissolution due to pruritus-inciting (pruriente) materia but without local swelling. One may say that if it is really pruritus that this describes, then the pain due to itching and the pain of ulceration are not different. The contrary of this statement is discussed by Galen, however, where he makes a clear distinction between "dolor pruriginosus" and "dolor ulcerosus." I believe these kinds of pain are different because in pruritus, while a continued dissolution of the skin is present, nevertheless this dissolution that causes pain is within the skin, for Avicenna said that the materia is contained between the two layers of the skin but that, in the pain of ulcers, the materia is not contained within the skin and produces not only a continual dissolution but also perforates the skin and produces the pain of ulceration. The reason why the skin is not ulcerated in pruritus is that the skin is denser and so does not permit the humors to pass through, but these, being confined, tear the tissues apart, thus producing continual dissolution and pain as a consequence.

From this discussion we understand that pruritus is a symptom of a damaged sense of touch, not damaged in every way, but perverted. This is what Galen taught, pointing out that although any symptom appertains to some morbid condition, this is related to two: to a particular disease, because humors abound where they should not, and to a morbid condition of an undetermined kind.

It may be objected that I err in calling pruritus a kind of pain, for, as Plato said, pruritus brings about a pleasurable sensation from scratching, and Socrates, as he scratched his shackled legs, said that he had never experienced greater delight. I reply that even if some pleasurable sensation appears in pruritus, this is not because of the pruritus but because of the scratching. Prior to the scratching, pain is indeed manifest. This is because, as we have said, the materia within the skin tears it apart, provokes dissolution of its continuity, and necessarily induces pain, in the scratching of which pleasurable sensation results because of the evacuation of the dolorific (pain-producing) materia. Therefore pleasurable sensation is perceived, as in other evacuations. Greater delight appears in scratching because evacuation is sudden and through many orifices. Thus the pleasure exists on account of the evacuation of humors, not on account of the pruritus.

In pruritus the greatest pain appears after scratching, for two reasons. First, as a result of the activity itself and the friction, new humors are brought to the site, distend the parts, and produce pain by forcing them apart. Secondly, the humors that cause itching are considerably inflamed by rubbing, so that the milder portion of the humors departs as a vapor while the more acrid remains, now causing pain and even greater itching from its expulsion.

I think experience shows that pruritus is invariably intensified by scratching. The reason why scabies (scabious disease) so frequently follows pruritus is because the humor is aggravated by scratching even to the point of producing sores. Thus it is understandable that the correct medicine for pruritus is not to scratch, if possible.

The immediate and material causes, as Galen taught, are excrements that are phlegmatic, nitrous, salty, and irritating. He gave for example nettles, quills, brine, and sea water, all of which cause pruritus. He distinguished between the materia of pruritus and that of scabies and lepra, saying that the former is a juice that is thin, salty, and stagnant, while the latter is a juice that is copious, salty, thick, and stagnant. Paullus, in following Galen, said that pruritus comes from decaying, somewhat salty phlegm, but not from bile. Avenzoar, who followed both Paullus and Galen, was of the same opinion, that scabies, which he called "vesicae" (blisters, not "vesiculae") comes from a thick and viscid humor, while pruritus, he said, comes from a sharp, thin humor.

Here the question arises as to whether the materia that causes pruritus is thinner than that which makes scabies. On the one hand is the authority of Galen, all the Greeks, and Avenzoar, who agreed that the juices of pruritus are the thinner. On the other hand is the argument that because, if the humor in pruritus does not get out as it does in scabies, then, it would seem, the humor that does not leave the skin would become the thicker. This reasoning is mostly on the authority of Avicenna, who distinguished between pruritus and scabies, saying that in pruritus there are no papulopustular lesions (bothor) just like those in scabies, and he adduced the argument that the materia of scabies is thinner, more fluid, and less deviated toward saltiness. It is clear that he felt that scabies comes from a thinner humor. Nearly all the Arabs, Serapion, Haly Abbas, and others, concurred with Avicenna.

To resolve this controversy, I would decide in accord with Galen that pruritus comes only from materia and humors that are rather thin. The argument that seems to contradict this view, namely that in pruritus the materia does not get out, is easy to dispose of. The reason why it does not leave is not because it is thicker but because the skin is condensed, so that the liquid, however fluid, cannot get out. That the skin has indeed been condensed in pruritus is seen in the lucid testimony of Galen, who wrote that in pruriginous conditions the skin of the body undergoes condensation. Furthermore, because the humors are not expelled in pruritus, another causative factor was adduced by Avicenna: the weakness of the expulsive power, which, he said, explains why the elderly, in whom the expulsive power is infirm and weak, cannot expel the humors from the skin.

Galen seems to have thought, however, that there is another cause for pruritus in old people. The excrements that excite pruritus have difficulty in evacuating through the skin, which is condensed and compacted by the chilled habitus of the body, so that excrements that are retained come forth thicker and, on further putrification, cause pruritus.

As to Avicenna's judgment, I say his head was exceedingly mixed up, for in the beginning he said one thing, and in the end and in the middle he said something different. Be that as it may, we can say that his view was peculiar to the Arabs and quite incorrect, while Galen's was right. In pruritus the skin may be torn apart, but we never see the emanation of a thick liquid, such as occurs in scabies. From this observation it is quite apparent that these humors and thick liquids are not abundant in pruritus.

It still may be asked why more pain appears and why it lasts longer in pruritus than in scabies. If the materia in pruritus were thicker, it would be easily explained as being due simply to the thickness of the materia. But if the materia of pruritus is thinner, it would not seem easy to give a reason. I will offer two explanations. First, it is simply not true that pain or distress are more intense or last longer in pruritus, because we frequently see the opposite, namely that in scabies itching is greater and more enduring. This being true, I say that worse itching may occur, but is less enduring, in scabies because the thick materia penetrates to the innermost parts and therefore produces greater pain and itching. Furthermore this materia, even if it is thick, nevertheless does get out of the skin, is markedly dispersed (difflatur), and hence is not enduring. Because the materia in pruritus is thin and does not penetrate the skin and flesh so intimately, it does not produce so much itching. That the thin materia is retained rather than expelled explains why the condition remains within the skin longer.

Now we turn to the immediate and material causes of pruritus. The mediate causes are several. First, the temperature of the body is concerned. The body that is hot and dry, or for some time hot and moist, is subject to pruritus. Age, too, is among the mediate causes, for the young and the old are especially susceptible to pruritic conditions, as Hippocrates wrote. The strongest factor among the causes is the manner of living, as we learn from Galen. If the body is dirty (lit abounds in sordes), and not kept clean, or if one often overloads the stomach and follows a bad diet, then one is apt to contract this kind of disease. Avicenna rightly said that those who eat sweet, salty, and bitter foods take pruritic diseases readily.

The diagnostic features of pruritus are quite clear. The whole body itches, and when it is scratched nothing comes from it but some scales or small flakes. The features that indicate the material causes are various. Avenzoar wrote that if pruritus comes from a burned out melancholic or acrid humor, some vestige of blackness will be apparent in the flesh. If it comes from blood, the disease will end sooner, even though it may be spread more widely throughout the body because blood is dispersed throughout the body. When pruritus results from a bilious and acrid humor, severe distress results, sharper and more pruritic, with a highly pleasurable sensation from scratching. Paullus rightly added that each humor causing pruritus may be diagnosed by the region of involvement, the temperature of the body, the age, the dietary habits, and the way of life of the patient. As these features indicate one humor or another, so they indicate one cause or another.

As to prognosis, indeed it may be said that pruritus rarely becomes chronic, for it degenerates into scabies. Even in recent cases pruritus often changes into scabies. Paullus and Avicenna said pruritus in old people can be relieved but never cured, but this is not always true, for I saw the celebrated octogenarian, Leonellus Pius, relieved of the most severe pruritus by means of medications. While it is rare for decrepit old people to be cured, nevertheless they are, sometimes. Hippocrates wrote that in patients wasting with illness, if pruritus causes suppression of the bowels, it will prove fatal. Avenzoar, too, described pruritus associated with severe tenesmus as the worst of all as regards restlessness and revulsion from food, because it is from cholera.

Next we consider the treatment, regarding which two important points must be clarified. First, salty and bitter humors must be removed from the body completely, and, secondly, regeneration of these humors must be guarded against. Their redevelopment will be prevented if the liver, a kind of factory for them, is adjusted and if the materia from which they are made is restrained. Since this materia comes from the way of life, the most important and effective means of cure lies in its correction. Thus one must choose air tempered with respect to its active quality, for in its passive quality it hastens the moist condition. Heat stimulates the humors more, while cold condenses the skin, thereby promoting pruritus considerably. Perturbations of the mind should be avoided. Exercises are harmful in pruritus, especially prior to purgation of the body, for, as Hippocrates and Theophrastus said, exercising unclean bodies makes ulcers. Rubbing and scratching should likewise be avoided.

A moderate and quiet life and plenty of sleep are helpful for two reasons. First, because, while one is asleep, itching is not aggravated by scratching, and secondly, during sleep the humors are better regulated by nature. Avicenna objected to sexual activity, and with justification, because, as he said, this sort of agitation excites vapors that are warm and harmful to the skin. In the skin these subsequently undergo decay, thereby increasing the saltiness, and this in turn increases the pruritus. Good elimination (alvum solutum) is also beneficial. If the bowels do not move spontaneously, they should be moved by clysters (enemas) or by brodia (broths). Among other things, it is helpful to keep the body clean, both by frequent changes of underclothing and linens and by baths, protecting the body from every kind of dirt and filth.

It is doubtful whether any kind of bath is helpful in pruritus. Paullus of Aegina apparently recommended the plain water bath. Avicenna said that a suitable bath is ordinary sea water, either not heated or warmed a little. Hippocrates, too, told of a certain Athenian, not relieved of pruritus by the efforts of any physician, who took the warm baths of the Island of Melos and by these, said Hippocrates, was completely cured of itching, but who later developed dropsy and died. Thus, on the one hand, according to Paullus, baths ought to be of fresh water, on the authority of Hippocrates and Avicenna, natural baths are more helpful.

To resolve this question I say that baths may be given in two ways, either prior to purgation simply to cleanse away the dirt and moisten the body, or after purgation to dry up the humors in the skin. If the baths are used for the former purpose, Paullus' view should doubtless be preferred, for fresh water cleanses better than the sea water so highly praised by Avicenna, or any other kind of water. We have here, too, the authority of Homer, who had Nausicaa wash her clothing, not in the sea, but in a river. Also plain water moistens quite well, or, as Paullus put it, plain water is "sysikmon to pathos," that is, it is "moistened with difficulty" (hard to make wetter).

Since the job of humectation (moistening) is to be done prior to purgation, plain water baths are preferable. After purgation, the salt baths and natural baths recommended by Avicenna are helpful, for after the body has been purged within, then the humors remaining in the skin are easily drained off. As for Hippocrates' case, it must be said that this outcome resulted from the improper use of water, because it undoubtedly extinguished the native heat in the same way that, as Aristotle said, dropsy sometimes comes from drinking wine.

The food should be of the best juices, cool, moist, and somewhat thick. Sweet, acrid, salty, and bitter foods should be avoided, as well as all oils and things like olive oil, regarding which Avicenna said, they interfere with digestion of foods and are easily inflamed. Averroes added that oil easily changes into something of a sulfurous nature, so he strongly objected to it, especially for frying.

Among the herbs, Avenzoar recommended lettuce and vinegar. In treating my patients, I usually have them eat lettuce, both in soups and with vinegar, every day at breakfast and supper. Avicenna especially recommended Indian melons, portulaca, borage, acid fruits, and even whole grains. The best meats are those of the kid and chicken because, as Avicenna and Galen said, this kind of meat adjusts defective and bitter humors. Chondrus, or grits (alica), made of farrago and ptisan, too, are very helpful. In regard to chondrus, Galen said that by its well known gelatinous quality (lentor) it adjusts and corrects the bitterness and deformity of the humors.

Here attention should be called to the fact that everything the sufferer from pruritus eats should be boiled rather than baked or fried, for fried and baked foods contain a humor or juice that is rather bitter, while foods that have been boiled do not. Not without justification the Latin physician, Theodorus Priscianus, said that foods for the patient with pruritus should be semiliquid (sorbiles, lit able to be sucked up). As to beverages, simply boiled water, barley water, or even a mild, thin, white wine would be suitable.

After the dietary regimen has been established, we turn to the purgation of the humors. First we consider whether the liver is feverish and whether the blood is overabundant. In either case purgation should begin with bloodletting. In fever of the liver, the blood should be taken from the vena iecoralis and, in overabundance of the blood, from the vena communis. But something always to be done before blood is removed is to loosen the bowels, either with a clyster or with cassia (senna), tamarind, or electuary of sebesten.

When the bowels have been loosened and the blood let, then the humors should be purged. If they are salty, acrid, or even rather thin, they should be cooled, adjusted, and brought to moderation. For preparing the humors, the following syrup is appropriate. Take 1 handful of portulaca, lettuce, borage, and endive and ½ ounce of Damascus prunes. Make a decoction in the usual manner. Take 4 ounces of this mixture and 1 ounce each of syrup of borage and syrup of fumitory, and mix.

After the humors have been prepared, they should finally be evacuated. For this purpose, rhubarb, thyme, senna, polypody, and black myrobalan are appropriate. This is indeed the place for polypody, which is the very best agent for evacuating the humors that cause scabies and pruritus.

If a bolus is desired, take 3 drams of Hamech's confection, 1 dram of finely powdered rhubarb, and 1 ounce of diacatholicon. Mix and make a bolus. If a draught is wanted, the following is useful. Take 4 scruples of rhubarb, infused and expressed in the usual manner, 3 ounces of syrup of polypody, and 4 ounces of a decoction of sebesten, tamarind, and black myrobalan in equal parts. Mix and make a potion.

Because the humor is often stubborn and rebellious, our purgation may be insufficient, so repetitions are frequently necessary. In this case, if it is believed to be of value, bleeding may perhaps be repeated, because sometimes after repeated purgation bleeding alone has cured the pruritus, as I have often observed.

After purgation, fomentations of endive or chicory juice are used to adjust the liver. I have not rejected these, but by far the most valuable of all is whey, not plain but, for treating pruritus, altered in the following way. Take 1 pound of goat's milk whey, 1 dram of black myrobalan, bruised and crushed by hand, and 1½ drams of thyme. This is allowed to stand overnight, then expressed, and taken in the morning 4 hours before eating. Whey so prepared adjusts the fever of the liver and relieves its obstruction, and any abnormal humor that remains in it is easily expelled. We can give whey by itself, but large quantities would be needed. It should be given every other morning, or even every day, more or less, according to the amount required.

After all these things have been attended to, we turn to local medication, to the agents that can dry out (exsiccate) the humors in the skin. Sulfur baths and sea water baths are now commendable. Because some patients are averse to baths, or baths may not be readily available, there are other medicaments for relieving pruritus. I have tried one used by both Oribasius and Paullus. It is made as follows. Take 4 ounces of lupine meal and 2 ounces of powdered sulfur, steep in vinegar, and rub vigorously over the whole body.

There are other medicines, such as, for example, powdered hellebore of either kind (black or white). Parsley (apium) is commendable, and pellitory (perdicium). After these herbs are gathered and dried, they are rubbed on the body.

I have another preparation I often use if the first is not successful. Take 1 ounce each of large rancid nuts and sulfur, and this, after levigating and macerating in parlsey juice, is rubbed on. Galen recommended acorn shells (recrementa balanorum) and said that a mixture of garum, sulfur, and oil is a simple and marvelous cure. It is to be noted, however, that whenever such powders are rubbed on, baths of plain water should always be given afterward. I usually recommend that the applications be made in a sweat room and that the bath be given immediately afterwards.

BOOK TWO, CHAPTER FOUR

ON SCABIES (THE SCABBY DISEASE)

SINCE SCABIES is quite closely related to pruritus and differs only somewhat, this chapter logically follows upon the preceding one. The disease was called "psora" by the Greeks. Avenzoar called it vesicular pruritus. Nearly all the Arabs called it scabies. Paullus of Aegina, in defining the disease, said that it is a roughness of the skin along with itching and a liquefication of the body, in varied forms, from which emanate certain little branny particles. Here it is to be noted that Actuarius practically copied these words from Paullus, but Actuarius' text does not read "little particles of bran emanate from scabies." Thus one must say either the manuscript of Paullus or of Actuarius is defective. I rather think that the manuscript of Paullus is erroneous, because almost no author among the Greeks, Arabs, or Latins said that little particles of bran occur in scabies. Indeed, as Galen said, in scabies and mild lepra there occurs shedding as from an old snake. He said this was called branny (furfuraceous) by Hippocrates in the sense of blister (vesica), a definition found in the teachings of Archigenes, according to Aetius.

Julius Pollux, judging from the various medical opinions, said "psorzn" is a particular ulcerative affection of the skin, reddish and with efflorescences in it. Cornelius Celsus seems to have described it somewhat differently. He said that scabies occurs with a rather firm and reddish swelling of the skin, in which pustules appear, sometimes moist, sometimes dry; and from these a kind of discharge comes, producing a pretty much continuous, itchy, ulcerative condition that spreads, in some patients quickly, in others slowly, in some cases dying out, and in others relapsing in a year or so. Here one must note, as we shall consider fully when we discuss the lichens, that according to Cornelius Celsus, true scabies is not the disease that some call "scabies" (the scabby disease), but is different. However, the other Greek and Arabic authors agreed upon the name, "scabies."

As to the material cause of this condition, I find a not wholly insignificant controversy between the Greek and Arabic writers. Galen wrote that scabies is a melancholic affection because it originates from materia of a melancholic nature. In another place, too, he said that scabies is due to melancholic juices, juices that are earthy and thick. Thus Galen seems consistently to have held the view that scabies comes from melancholic materia and juices. On the other hand, Avicenna said that the materia of scabies is sanguineous, either melancholic or phlegmatic-salty. One gathers from Avicenna that the materia of scabies is sanguineous and full of various qualities, not only melancholic but also salty and phlegmatic. Serapion, not the least credible of the Arabs, was of the opinion that scabies comes from thick, decadent, sanguineous material. Haly Abbas attributed it to a mixture of salty phlegm and bilious blood. Actuarius seems to have followed the opinion of the later Greeks, for he said that scabies comes from a mixture of all the humors.

In this controversy, I think one must say that two kinds of scabies occur, one dry, the other moist. The variety in which either nothing exudes or in which something thick, earthy, and dry is exuded, I call dry. The moist form, on the other hand, is that in which sanious, moist, thin, and bitter material exudes, or else thick, foul material. If we speak only of the dry type, surely it comes from a superabundance of melancholic juices, and even if other humors contribute to the generation of this type of scabies, nevertheless the greater part of its materia is melancholic. This can be recognized easily by the color, since patients suffering with this dry scabies always show livid and dark sores and stigmata. When Galen said that scabies is a melancholic affection, he was thinking of dry scabies, and he recognized the condition as melancholic through superabundance, which is to say, the greater part of the effectuating materia is melancholic. Thus both Galen and those who followed him were speaking of the dry type when they said scabies is a melancholic affection.

In speaking of all kinds of scabies, both the dry and the moist, the Arabs and those who followed them have rightly stated that it comes from all kinds of humors, not only the thick and dry ones, but also the thin and moist. Indeed if we observe the generation of moist scabies, surely salty phlegm brings it about. Both kinds of bile also contribute, and sometimes a bilious ichor, and sometimes all of these humors.

Thus it was rightly said by the Arabs that scabies is a complex of every humor in proportion to its moistness or dryness. What do we say of Avicenna's belief that every kind of scabies comes from the sanguineous humor? I say he was right, because the materia of scabies is always sanguineous because scabies is an affection involving the entirety of the body, and no other humor is spread throughout the entire body as the blood is by the circulation (ambitu). But the blood that produces scabies is not pure. It is thick, sometimes salty because of decay or because of its mixture with bile. Sometimes it is irritating, as it is whenever melancholic. It suffices to say that in scabies blood is always to blame.

The primitive (predisposing) causes are multiple, and foremost is the age of youth and childhood, because individuals at this period are indiscreet in their diet, eat the greatest amount of food, and produce the greatest amount of excrement. From heat and exertion the blood turns more bitter so that in these age groups the materia for scabies is especially abundant. Leisure, too, promotes scabies, for the recrements are not discharged but are held in the skin. Decaying in the flesh, they turn bitter, making ulcers and giving rise to scabies. Unseasonable exercises, that is, those engaged in with impure body and diet, are apt to make scabies because, as Galen noted, the defective humors hidden in the body are brought to the surface, and, unable to escape from the skin, they are retained, undergo decay, and produce scabies. Not without reason the divine Hippocrates said exercising an impure body makes ulcers.

Indifference and neglect are apt to produce scabies. People who do not change their clothes or wash off dirt are quite liable to the affection because the filth retained on the surface acquires bitterness that later produces scabies. Quintus Serenus, a most ancient and weighty physician, explained this nicely:

> Often it is that sweat unwashed and food unworthy
> Incite the evils of the grievous itch.

The fact that poor juices and poor food readily induce scabies was quite clearly indicated by Galen. The bad foods are the salty ones, such as meats and fishes, and the bitter and acrid ones, such as onion, garlic, and leeks. Thus the poor are frequently afflicted with scabies, since they eat this kind of diet. Sweets readily make scabies, for as Galen said, they all tend to inflame the spleen and liver, and this increases the inflammation.

The time of year may be listed among the causative factors, according to Avicenna, who said that dry scabies occurs in the autumn and the moist in the winter because melancholy abounds in the autumn, inducing dry scabies, and in the winter, the phlegm in fact is salty, and the result is scabies. Seneca, too, wrote that certain kinds of water convey scabies into the body, particularly that which comes from dew. Such water, Plutarch said, causes lepra.

Galen said that there are some women who through their peculiar nature are prone to accumulate excrements that readily instigate scabies. Thus it appears Galen included a natural disposition among the primitive causes of the disease.

Contagion is among the causes, for Galen, reviewing certain kinds of diseases acquired by contagion, listed scabies among them. How the contagion comes about Alexander explained satisfactorily. He said scabies is contagious because of a kind of viscid, sticky moisture which emanates from the surface, adheres in that region of the body, and is easily communicated from one body to another. Here one should observe that transmission by contagion is a feature of moist scabies and that, while dry scabies can be so taken, this is infrequent.

"An act of God" (motus criticus naturae, an action chosen by nature) is among the causes. Sometimes certain acute diseases, not terminating naturally through swellings or dissolutions, may go into scabies.

I may be asked how scabies is to be recognized when it occurs spontaneously and will go away as a result of natural phenomena. The recognition of spontaneous scabies, Hippocrates said, is based on the fact that when it develops in infants and children, it comes on gradually, and this kind of scabies does not come from other diseases. But when scabies develops after another disease and comes on suddenly, then it is not the spontaneous variety, and it arises, not gradually, but abruptly (per crisis).

The diagnostic features of scabies are the presence of pruritus, sometimes with ulceration of the skin, sometimes with the exudation of dry material or perhaps material that is somewhat moist. Scabies differs from pruritus, in which there is no discharge; yet something, dry or moist, does exude in scabies.

Concerning the recognition of the types of scabies, much has been handed down from the Arabic medical writers. They said that if scabies comes from corrupted blood, the pruritus will be mild and not disagreeable, and moisture will be seen, accompanied by pustules that are pointed and not very broad. No fissures will be present, and no pain, and the color will tend to be light red or pale. Quickly there will develop discharges that are copious and soon laudable. When the disease comes from phlegm, the pruritus will be not very intense, but it will be unpleasant. The color will tend to be livid, and much moisture will appear, along with thicker and broader pustules, and when these dry up and are scratched, there will come away something like dry, parched scales. Much discharge will be produced rather late in the course of the disease. When scabies comes from salty phlegm, the pruritus will be more intense, and the color will tend to be bluish. When it comes from bile, the pruritus will be much sharper and more severe, and the pustules more pointed and drier, and if anything comes from them it will be a drier material, or bilious and ichorous, and the color of the skin will be pallid or whitish. When it comes from a melancholic humor, the Arabs said the pruritus is milder and rather deeply seated, but without discharge, and if anything comes forth, it will be small in quantity, thick, and only slightly irritant. The color will be ashen, reddish brown, or dark.

When I said that according to the Arabs the pruritus of the melancholic type is slight, there may be some question, for Galen wrote that both scabious and leprous patients have more severe pruritus than others, and, not relieved by scratching, they tear themselves to pieces. He said that this is because thick, viscid, and sticky humor stubbornly hangs on within the skin, and that it can be eradicated by ointments only with great effort. If Galen's opinion is correct, then the melancholic type of scabies causes extreme pruritus, for, as we have said, scabies is a melancholia due to superabundance and therefore causes great itching. Hence the pruritus is intense, the Arabs' opinion to the contrary notwithstanding.

I would say that when the Arabs spoke of melancholic scabies as being not accompanied by great and intense pruritus, they were thinking of the melancholic humor as least acrid and irritating, which is quite natural, but when Galen said it is a melancholic affection, meaning it is a melancholia by superabundance, he meant that along with the melancholic humor there may be salty phlegm and bile too. Then because of the tenacity of the melancholic humor, the irritant bile and salty phlegm make the itching unmitigable.

As to the prognosis in scabies, little is to be said. What Plato wrote should not be passed by in silence, that in scabies and pruritus there is more pain than satisfaction in scratching, for what is within seethes and swells (gliscit) and cannot be got out by rubbing, which reaches only the irritated surface.

In view of the foregoing, we may presume that scabies, however painful it is, may nevertheless afford sensual pleasure (voluptatem). It is never actually dangerous but, on the contrary, it may save a great many individuals from a number of impending diseases.

Avicenna wrote that scabies comes from a humor that is quite sharp, harsh, and bulky, and in it the pustules are more acuminate when they are numerous, since the warm, sharp materia spreads widely and disseminates in numerous fragments. Thus when it is more widespread deep in the skin, it is due to materia that is not so harsh and sharp.

Scabies has the peculiarity of affecting males by predilection, especially physicians, as Galen said. Another feature is that of being transformed readily into lepra unless it is cured. Thus we must be earnest in learning about its treatment, which in part is the same as that of pruritus and in part has its own particular methods.

The diet is much the same as for pruritus in that nearly all the things helpful in the one are helpful in the other. A peculiar point concerns pork, to which, Plutarch wrote, the Jews and foreigners are averse because these people are highly susceptible to scabies. Swine do suffer from this condition.

As to treatment, Paullus warned that one must above all judge whether the whole body is involved. If so, he considered bloodletting necessary at once, but always, before this is done, the bowels must be evacuated. Blood should be let mainly from the right side because the liver is rarely affected in scabies. I say rarely because it may occur through contagion, but even so the liver is not necessarily involved.

Two questions arise here. First, why do I say, as Paullus did, that the vein should always be cut? It is because, as we have said, Avicenna considered the blood always to blame in scabies.

Secondly, if scabies is the result of a melancholic humor, as we have indicated, quoting Galen, it would seem that the blood should be let rather from the left side, because the spleen particularly is always affected in melancholic conditions, although, as we have said, blood should be drawn generally from the right side.

As to the first question, one must say in brief it is true that in scabies the blood is subjected to decayed humors, as Avicenna said. But he did not say that the blood is full of them. It is easy to see that this is true, for Avicenna looked to purgation in the treatment of scabies rather than venesection, as if he were quite sure that defective humors abound in the blood itself.

As to the second question, one may reply in either of two ways. For one thing, in the scabies of the Greeks, which always comes from melancholic humor, the spleen is always affected, hence the blood should be drawn from the left side. Alternatively, it may be replied that, while scabies is the result of melancholic humor, nevertheless the liver itself is affected primarily, for the melancholic humor is made, not in the spleen, but in the liver, which produces melancholic humor whether it burns with fever or is cold and dry.

You might ask how then can the spleen be considered adjunctive in the production of melancholic humor. This may occur in two ways. First, it does not attract and hold back the refuse of the blood the way it ought, on account of the excess of melancholic liquid in the rest of the body, which the spleen is said to produce. Alternatively, it attracts more than it should, for the spleen, when abnormally warm and dry, vigorously attracts blood that is full of refuse rather than clean blood. Such blood swells the spleen and is converted into melancholic juice by the body just as it is by the spleen. Hence we may believe that in a melancholic condition, and especially a scabious one, the liver is the primary source. So we are correct in saying that blood should be drawn from the right side.

After the blood has been drawn, the humors should be prepared with the following syrup or one like it. Take ½ handful each of leaves of fumitory, scabiosa, lupine, and borage. Make a decoction in the usual way. Take 4 ounces of this and 1 ounce each of syrup of fumitory and borage juice. Mix.

After preparation of the humors, we turn to purgation. For purging the melancholic humor in scabies Avicenna strongly recommended thyme, senna, polypody, black myrobalan, and citron, and to these we add rhubarb. In treating chronic scabies Avicenna thought highly of aloes, which, he said, is curative if taken frequently. Our syrup of polypody is especially effective in these conditions.

After purgation of the humors, we turn to the local medications. In ordering these, we use first the detergents because the skin is rough and must be cleansed, and secondly the medicines that purge the pores, which are clogged with pus and bloody corruption and have to be purged. Thirdly, we use the medicines that cut into the disease, because the humor that makes scabies is thick and viscid and needs a penetrative (incisive) medicine. Finally, the exsiccative medicines should be used because in scabies there are small, moist sores that need to be dried up.

Among the detergent agents Galen wrote about we may list barley meal, broad beans, pulse, lupine, and sweet almonds. Among those that cleanse the pores are nettle seeds, squill, iris (L, ? sword-lily), niter, saltpeter, abrotanum, and bitter almonds. Among the penetrants, the strongest is vinegar. Those that exsiccate and cleanse are both kinds of hellebore, scales of copper, lime, litharge, sulfur vivum, quicklime, and the like, which are compounded in the usual manner.

As to the composition and use of these, four points are to be observed. First, the medicines that remove scabies are usually painful. To eliminate this feature they should be mixed with such things as oil of roses, butter, or some fat like chicken fat, goose grease, or egg yolk. The second point concerns the agents for drying up scabies. The adstringent ones should be completely avoided. The reason, as given by Galen, is that adstringents do not interfere at all with things taken internally for cleaning out the passageways, but actually increase their strength because the internal passageways are wider, so that adstringents given internally cannot obstruct them. But medicines applied externally are different. Adstringents readily make narrow and occlude the external passages, as a result of which no pathway would remain open for other medicines. Thirdly, the topical medication for scabies should be applied in a warm place and on parts of the body that have been warmed; then they penetrate better. Thus the ancients usually did their anointing in the warm sunshine, in steam baths, or beside a fire, as we learn from Hippocrates. Fourthly, the medicines should be used only on alternate days because they penetrate quite deeply, and during the interval nature can work against the disease with the aid of the medication.

Medication good for the itching can be prepared as follows, or in a like manner. Take 1 dram each of both kinds of hellebore, 1½ drams of litharge, 1 ounce of rose oil, ½ ounce of fresh butter, and 5 drams of lupine meal. Mix carefully, and make a liniment. If a stronger one is desired, the following is typical. Take 1 dram each of niter and sulfur vivum. Wash three times in strong vinegar. Add ½ ounce of rose oil, 2 egg yolks, and ½ ounce of chicken fat. Mix, and make a liniment.

For getting rid of scabies, thermal baths are available, sulfurous waters especially being likely to cure it promptly, after the body has been purged.

It is worth considering whether quicksilver or sublimated silver (mercury) is appropriate. Avicenna and his followers recommended them as marvelous. The more recent vendors of medicines (L pharmacopolae, quacks) usually use this kind of medicine. On the other hand, we know that mercury is a poisonous and dangerous agent and therefore unsuitable. Even the Greeks do not mention it as a remedy. So I say in scabious conditions, if mild and recent, mercury should be entirely avoided. Great danger is involved of incorporating more of it than necessary or of using more of the ointment than is wise. Whenever a considerable hazard is involved, we must always avoid running a risk in any case that is not of itself dangerous. If the scabies were chronic and malignant, then we might use such medicines. They should be diluted, however, and mixed with milder things so that we should have less anxiety.

BOOK TWO, CHAPTER FIVE

ON LEPRA

RELATED to scabies is another condition commonly known as "lepra." In this the materia is the same as in scabies, according to not only Galen but also Oribasius, Paullus, and all the authorities. Paullus defined the condition as a roughness of the skin with itching, a condition that liquefies (colliquatione) the body from a melancholic humor, consumes the deep parts of the body in small rings, and causes the shedding of scales like those of fishes.

As to this definition, one may note that Paullus said it is a harshness of the skin with pruritus and colliquation. We have it from Aetius that Archigenes considered lepra to be different from leuce and alphos, which are varieties of vitiligo. Lepra is rough to the touch and induces itching. Since only the skin is affected and is excoriated, the layers beneath appear to be healthy. Hippocrates' view of the subject was that in lepra the skin is thick because it is permeated by a thick and viscid humor.

In leuce there is neither roughness nor itching, and if the skin (L cutis) is removed, the underlying flesh (L caro) looks spotted, whiter than normal, and if rubbed the skin itself or the flesh beneath becomes reddish immediately. This is true particularly if the case is of the curable kind. The lesions of alphos, however, are not pruritic and are not rough, although macules appear that closely resemble scales. Archigenes said too that lepra differs from scabies in that sometimes minute branny flakes come from the lesions.

In lepra the scales are like those of large fish; indeed the body desquamates in this condition. Julius Pollux in defining lepra said that there are many impetiginous lesions, rough, ulcerative, sometimes reddish or quite red, and sometimes of a pale hue, and that these are hard to cure. He added that in lepra the nails are diseased, a distinction to be noted. That famous physician, Actuarius, seemed to be of about the same opinion as the other Greeks when he said that lepra is called "apo ton lepidon," or "derived from scales," although the scholiast Nicander said that the name lepra comes rather from "apo ton lepruneathai," which means "to be made scabby and become white." The Aldine edition of the Greek text mistakenly reads "lepuneothai."

The Greeks all agreed that lepra is, as it were, a kind of scabies, deformed and "magnam" (large, grand, important, in this 1572 text; "nigram," black, grievous, deadly, in the 1623 text). They agreed with Galen that the materia of lepra is a juice that is melancholic, while Archigenes seems to have added that it is also viscid and thick. Galen apparently confirmed this in stating that lepra and scabies result from an abundant, thick, salty, stagnant humor, just as if he had said that lepra comes from phlegm mixed with salt, provided that the melancholic juice is always dominant. This "lepra of the Greeks" has been so called by the Arabs, particularly by Avicenna. He described two varieties of albara, white and dark, clearly interpreting black albara as being the lepra Graecorum. He said, among other things, that black albara is an excoriated and scabious impetigo that attacks and irritates the skin violently and causes scaling and itching because of the melancholic humor that the skin imbibes. The whole nature and picture of lepra Graecorum is expressed by these words, which it is perfectly clear came from Serapion, from whom Avicenna undoubtedly borrowed them.

Thus I wonder at Tagautius and others, who wrote effusively on this subject but seemed never to have actually hit upon the point. I wonder even at Haly Abbas, who alone of the Mauritanian authors seems in manifest error to have called lepra the leuce of the Greeks and the white albara of Avicenna. Lepra is black albara, not white.

One must recognize what Avicenna understood by the name "lepra." His view clearly was that it is actually the elephantiasis of the Greeks, which is a kind of swelling of the entire body. Even nowadays elephantiasis is called lepra. It was a patient with this disease, the most difficult one to cure, whom Christ, our Lord, cured. Thus lepra as described by Avicenna and Avenzoar is the elephantiasis Graecorum, and the lepra Graecorum is the black albara of Avicenna.

Some, following Celsus, have considered lepra to be a kind of scabies, but I am of the opinion that it is rather the impetigo of Celsus, who described four varieties of scabies. In all of them, he said, scaling occurs.

To put it briefly, the lepra of the Greeks, the black albara of Avicenna, and the impetigo of Cornelius Celsus are one and the same. That this is so is seen perfectly easily and clearly in the words of Celsus, who said his impetigo involves the nails, which, as we pointed out above, occurs in lepra, according to Julius Pollux.

This affection is classified as a disease involving roughness and smoothness. The internal and material cause is predominantly the melancholic humor. The efficient cause is an imbalance of the liver, the spleen, or both. As to the primary and procatarctic causes, we must repeat what we said about scabies, for in Galen's opinion both conditions come from the same causes. Averroes wrote what Avicenna had said previously, that lepra takes its origin from heredity and from coitus with a menstruating woman. While this is to be understood of the lepra of the Arabs, that is, elephantiasis, it is also true of the lepra of the Greeks. This disease, as Galen wrote, is peculiar to older people, so age must be given a place among the primary causes, as Hippocrates too classified the melancholic diseases.

It may be asked whether lepra results from contagion, for Galen wrote that psora is, and lepra is a deformed type of psora, as we have hitherto said, so it might be even more contagious. But Alexander of Tralles wrote that lepra is not contagious and said that in both vitiligo and lepra the humors are viscid, thick, and earthy rather than catching (L adhaerere, lit sticky). Aristotle was of the opinion that lepra is not contagious, although Petrus Apponensis seems to have held otherwise.

As to this controversy I judge that all forms of lepra, that of the Greeks as well as that of the Arabs, are contagious. Indeed Avicenna in reviewing the various causes of lepra said that it may be acquired both by contagion from infected air and by proximity to a leprous individual, which is what Avenzoar also wrote. As to Alexander's opinion, I say that either the text is corrupt or by lepra Alexander meant the black alphos, the same as Haly Abbas meant by leuce. I am obliged to think this for a number of reasons. First, Alexander described lepra and leuce as being alike. But the lepra of the Greeks is completely dissimilar from leuce, although alphos is quite similar. Alexander said, too, that lepra is not contagious because the humor is in the surface and nothing comes out of the skin. But in lepra Graecorum there is always an exudation of some humor, and this is another reason for saying that true lepra

Graecorum should not have been what Alexander meant.

As to Aristotle, I reply that he did not expressly say that lepra is not contagious but that it is less contagious than psora, a fact we can confirm because the materia is more earthy. Or we might say that, according to Aristotle, by the name lepra is to be understood vitiligo, i.e., alphos, for, as it appears, according to the school of Nicander, "lepra" was used by the Greeks for any abnormal whiteness of the skin, just as "alphos" was "oi pos ten lepreoesthai," which means, "to become white."

One thing I wish to say—and that will be enough—is that Plutarch stated that people who walk in woods heavy with dew contract lepra. This is because, as Laitus said, dew stings and excoriates the flesh or else because the dew that clings to the trees takes from them some kind of acrid corpuscular material that sticks to the body, excoriates it, and induces lepra. It is true that dew liquefies the body, as shown by the fact that fat women who get their clothes wet with it are much weakened. The geoponics (agriculturists) write that when cattle feed on vegetation heavy with dew, they become lean.

The diagnostic features of lepra are the same as those of psora. Lepra does have the peculiar feature of being scaly. The sweat is fetid, and few remedies work.

Prognostically, just as scabies goes into lepra, so lepra goes into elephantiasis. Cornelius Celsus said that lepra, like impetigo, responds poorly to treatment. There might well be some question as to how lepra can be converted into elephantiasis, for Galen in one reference plainly stated that elephantiasis changes into lepra, and he repeated the statement in another citation when he referred to the case of a philosopher with elephantiasis who became leprous after eating snake meat.

I reply that it is possible both for elephantiasis to change into lepra and lepra into elephantiasis, for if the humors that make lepra in the skin were to fill all the flesh, they would make elephantiasis; and so also if the humors that make elephantiasis when in the flesh were concentrated in the skin, they would make lepra. Thus the transition of one disease into the other is possible.

In Hippocrates' opinion, the easiest cases to cure are those involving the youngest patients, the cases more recent in onset, and those that involve the soft, fleshy parts of the body.

The treatment of this disease is the same as for scabies, for lepra differs from scabies only to a greater or lesser degree. As I have said, lepra is a deformed kind of scabies and so requires stronger medicine. Galen said that the agents helpful in lepra are the ones that are strongly drying, that strip the pores clean and purge them.

Numerous remedies are listed in the writings of various authors, but to save time I will not review them all. Cornelius Celsus gave two, originally from Protarchus and Serapion. Marcellus gave certain particular remedies such as herba Brittanica taken with food or drink, wolf dung rubbed in with vinegar, and smearing the patient with the blood of a mountain goat, all of which were recommended by Dioscorides. Among other agents, Galen spoke well of cantharides and stated that, while some authors removed the wings, feet, and heads, he used the insects whole. Hippocrates advised the removal of the wings, feet, and heads, and Galen did so in order to concur with him. It is important to know that, if cantharides is given internally, it must be diluted, as Hippocrates insisted. If used externally, the insects may be applied whole.

BOOK TWO, CHAPTER SIX

ON LICHENS

OF THE cutaneous affections, there is one other, called "lichen." A number of foreigners have called this "the serpiginous disease" or "zerna." Haly Abbas called it "petigo" and "sarpedo." The common name is "volatica" (L, witch).

The lichens, as Galen defined them, are a particular kind of rough lesions of the skin, as it were, accompanied by great itching, from which materia emanates. The Greeks and Arabs set up two classes of lichen, the one benign and mild, the other severe (ferum). Galen wrote that the severe varieties are those not benefited by agents of moderate drying power, but much irritated by exsiccatives. He described two kinds of impetigo, the benign and the severe. Avicenna wrote that one form of impetigo is moist and oozes dew when rubbed, and the other is dry. The moist variety is the healthier, while the dry comes from salty phlegm that changes into a melancholic humor. He went on to say that the latter form of impetigo excorticates because of extreme dryness and numerous deep extensions (profundationes). The former does not excorticate but stays in one place. The latter spreads and is malignant. Galen appears to have confirmed this when he wrote that one form of impetigo is acute, the other chronic.

From all this I presume that the scabies Cornelius Celsus described is none other than the lichen of the Greeks and the impetigo of the Arabs. It is quite certain that all impetiginous conditions were classed as lichens by the Greeks, and especially the severe form of scabies that Cornelius Celsus spoke about, which the Greeks called "agrian" because it is more itchy and harder to cure. It is true, we see, that the Greeks never called psora "agrian" but only the lichens.

It seems quite certain to me that the scabies of Celsus was the lichen of the Greeks. Thus I wonder why Tagautius, otherwise an accurate man, did not see this. He always said the psora of the

Greeks was the scabies of the Latins.

The materia of the lichens, according to the Greeks and Arabs, is a mixture of thin and watery humors with thick ones, a mixture in which the thick humor, or the thin one, or sometimes the fiery one, predominates. The disease involves the whole of the body, particularly the face and chin, as Galen wrote.

Lichen involving the chin, as Galen mentioned, is an especially miserable disease, inducing severe itching and tension of the affected parts. It is not a little dangerous, for it may spread over the whole face, sometimes involves the eyes, and may cause extreme ugliness.

It is doubtful whether lichen of the chin is the same as the "mentagra" that Pliny described. He said that during the reign of Tiberius Claudius Caesar (14-37 A.D.) it first appeared in Italy, carried in from Asia by the knight Perusinus.

Some think that lichen of the chin and mentagra are the same condition, for Pliny himself said that mentagra had been called lichen in the Greek nomenclature. I would refute this opinion for three reasons. First, lichen is a very old disease, as we learn from Hippocrates; Theophrastus (370-285 B.C.) too, mentioned lichen. It is impossible that this disease was new at the time of Pliny (23-79 A.D.). Secondly, according to Pliny, mentagra was painless and not dangerous to life. Galen, however, said that lichen of the chin was a dangerous disease, with itching and pain. Thirdly, Pliny said it was called lichen in Greek nomenclature as if the disease was different but was so called for want of another name. It would seem that mentagra attacked only men of prominence and did not affect women or slaves, but lichen of the chin is indifferent as to whom it affects. The stongest evidence that lichen of the chin and mentagra are distinct comes from Galen: where he mentioned mentagra, the Greek codex reads "melitagrae," one sees, although it ought to read "mentagrae." In that place Galen gave also a lengthy discussion of lichen of the chin, and so it is quite apparent that he made a distinction between them. Then too, Marcellus, a most painstaking (diligentissimus) physician, distinguished between mentagra and impetigo or lichen, for he wrote that Soranus the Physician became the most famous man in Aquitania by curing this condition.

The predisposing causes of impetigo or lichen are all those of scabies and lepra: a bad diet, the time of the year—in the spring, Hippocrates wrote—contagion, and the others.

The diagnostic features of this condition are the numerous sores of rounded form, within which an opening may occur, or sometimes broad plaques (platea) with itching, burning, and roughness. Sometimes from the affected part something like bark comes off. Infrequently moisture like sweat drips from it. The color may be reddish or pallid.

As for the prognosis in lichen, it often goes into scabies and lepra, as we have it from Galen, especially if neglected or not treated promptly, as it ought to be. Hippocrates wrote that the lichens are easier to cure in young patients and in the fleshy and softer parts of the body. Avicenna said that impetigo is cured more quickly when the thin materia exceeds the thick and when it is recent and mild rather than chronic and severe. Pollux, in speaking of lichen agrior (severe), said that it is rough, uneven, and indurated (dusiatos).

As to the treatment of the condition, little is to be said, for about the same regimen and other measures are helpful as in pruritus, and this we have described heretofore. The diet should be especially moistening, as Avicenna noted. Thus plain water baths are to be highly recommended. Serapion felt that acrid and salty foods are to be avoided and everything that promotes bilious juices. Especially objectionable are undiluted wine and dates and sexual excess. If blood abounds, the vein for draining the liver should be sectioned. Avicenna believed that leeches should certainly be applied, even if there were no indication for bloodletting. The humors should then be prepared and evacuated by the medicines for eliminating both watery and thick humors.

Following preparation and purgation, one turns to local agents, giving attention to the necessity for their being of more than one kind. When lichen comes from benign humors, the more benign agents will do, but if from more malignant humors, stronger and more potent medicines are appropriate. Galen said, too, the lichens that might change into psora and lepra require medicines that are potently exsiccative, cleansing, and effective in opening the passageways (meatus). Hippocrates wrote that the impetigines are best eliminated by vinegar and thus manna (see thus in glossary), pumice, sulfur with vinegar, burned wild cress (nasturtium), snake skin, and the root of wild sorrel. For mild lichen, the benign type described by Galen and Oribasius, I use the fasting saliva preferably of a child—this is a remedy women are familiar with. In bad cases, I use native sulfur tied in a linen bag and steeped in vinegar. Marcellus listed many remedies. Marking around impetigo with gold, he said, will cure it. Aelius Promotus, Democritus, and others spoke of a great many things, which anyone can look up in their writings. I am certainly not going over them one by one. I often obtain good results using sulfur with vinegar.

The four illustrations next following are from photographs provided in 1966 by E. Zoli, of Forli, Italy, whose photograph of the Forli Museum bust of Mercurialis is placed at the end of the Introduction.

The Abbey of San Mercurialis, Forli, where Hieronymus Mercurialis and members of his family are entombed.

The chapel in the Abbey of San Mercurialis where their bodies lie.

The Mercurialis tomb in the chapel. At the left is the inscription commemorating Johannus, the son of Hieronymus and Francesca Mercurialis.

Inscription on Mercurialis' Tomb.

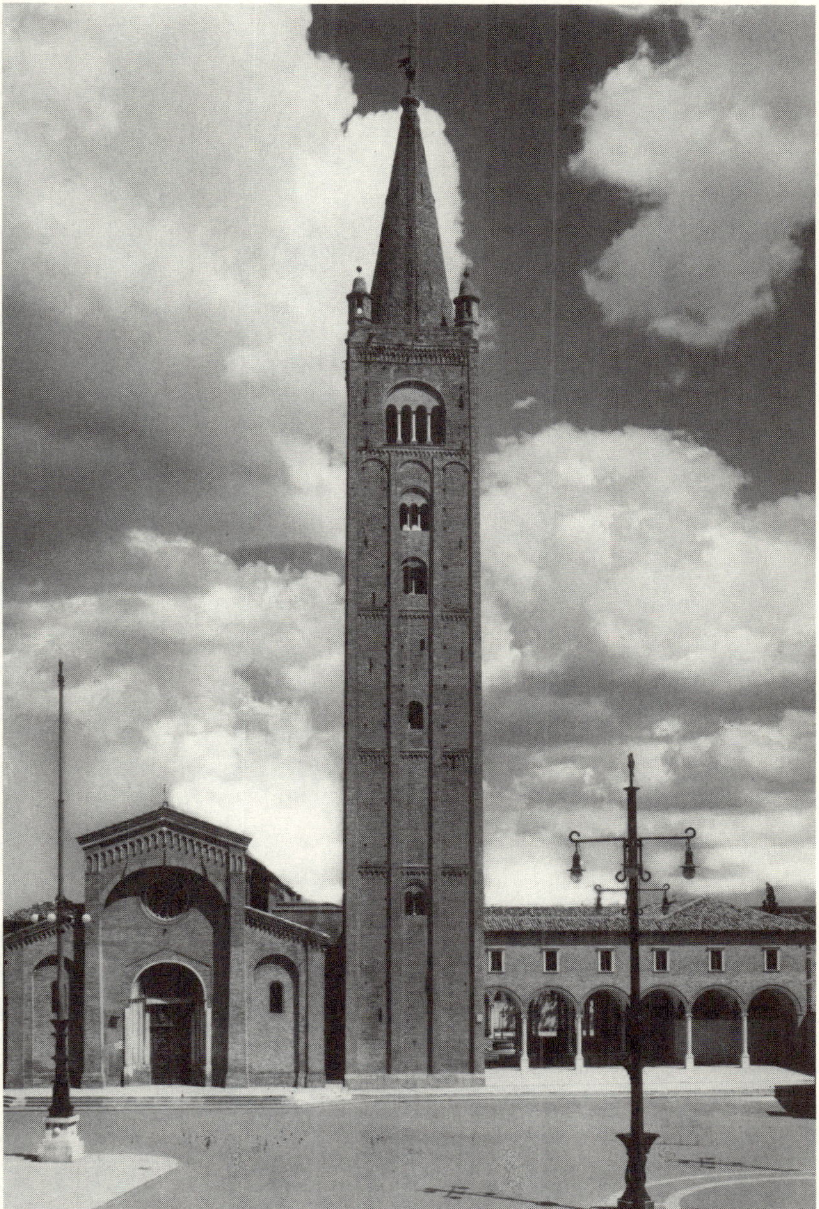

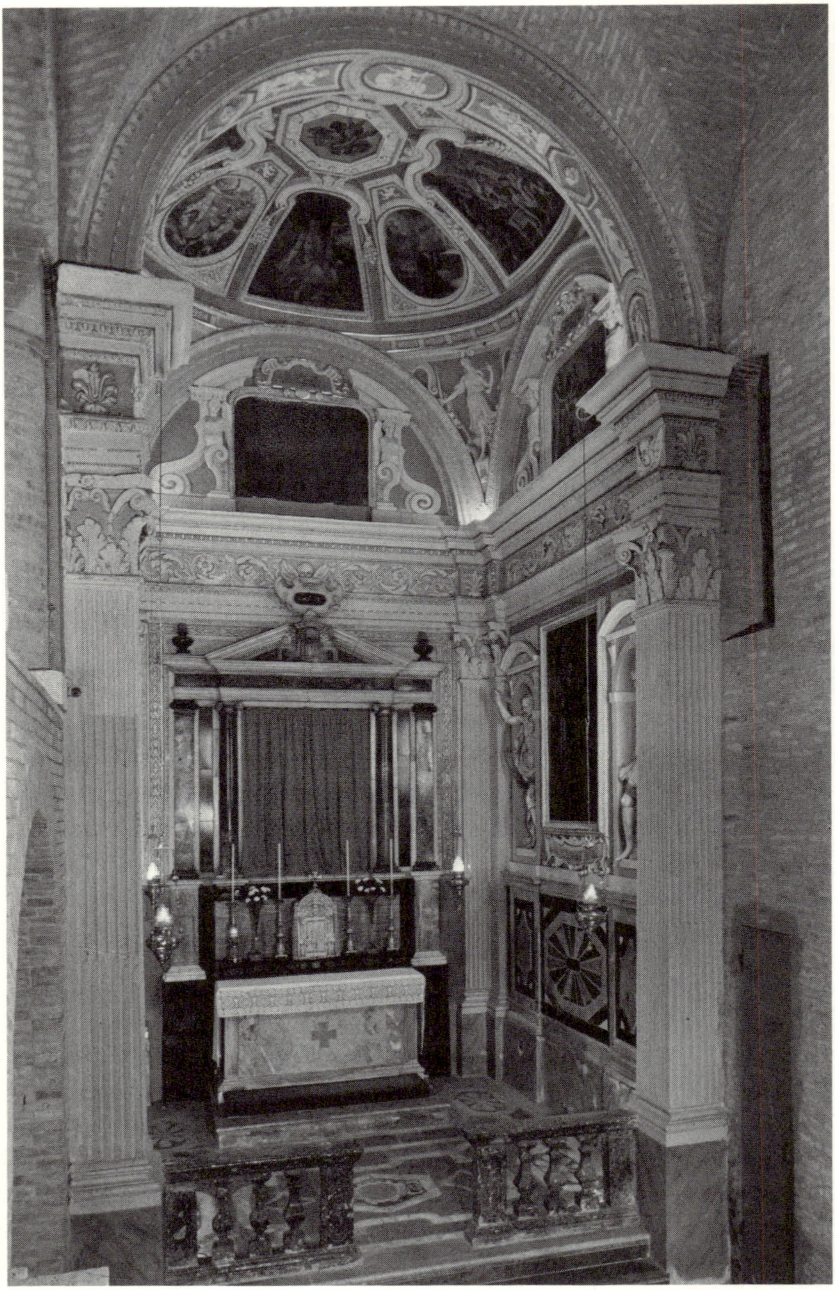

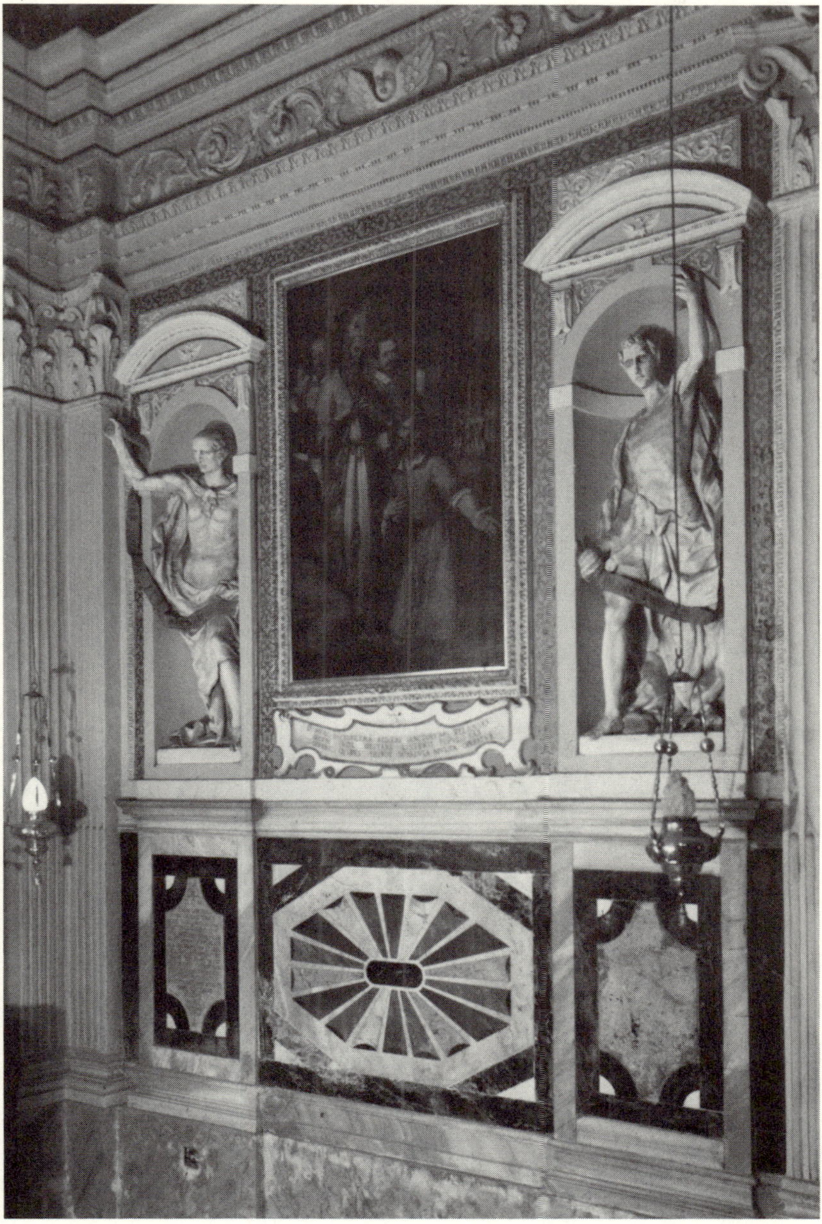

To the Lord Most Good, Most Great

This epigraph in memory of Johannus Mercurialis, a youth most pleasing to all because of his most gracious manner and the worthiness of his life, who, while pursuing studies in the well known Academy of Hispaniarus Salmanticus, died of a pestilential fever, has been erected by Hieronymus and Francesca Mercurialis for their beloved son, who lived twenty-five years and four months and died on the Ides of March (March 15) 1597.

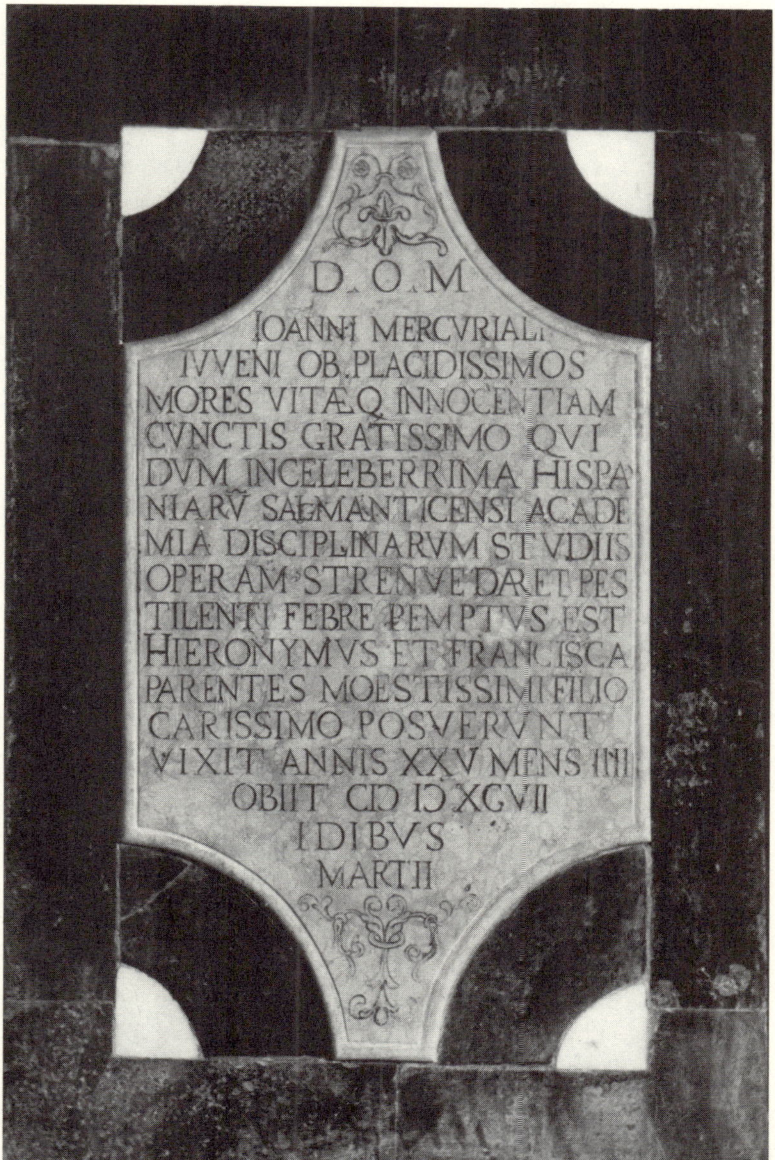
D. O. M
IOANNI MERCVRIALI
IVVENI OB PLACIDISSIMOS
MORES VITÆQ INNOCENTIAM
CVNCTIS GRATISSIMO QVI
DVM INCELEBERRIMA HISPA
NIARV SALMANTICENSI ACADE
MIA DISCIPLINARVM STVDIIS
OPERAM STRENVE DARET PES
TILENTI FEBRE PEMPTVS EST
HIERONYMVS ET FRANCISCA
PARENTES MOESTISSIMI FILIO
CARISSIMO POSVERVNT
VIXIT ANNIS XXV MENS IIII
OBIIT CIƆ IƆ XCVII
IDIBVS
MARTII

"The Return of Saint Mercurialis to Forli from Jerusalem," by Sante Tito (1536-1605), in the Abbey of St. Mercurialis, Forli. Hieronymus Mercurialis, a deacon, is depicted at the Saint's right, the painter, represented as a subdeacon, at his left. This illustration was provided by Dr. Walter Vichi of the Forli Institute of Arts and Culture.

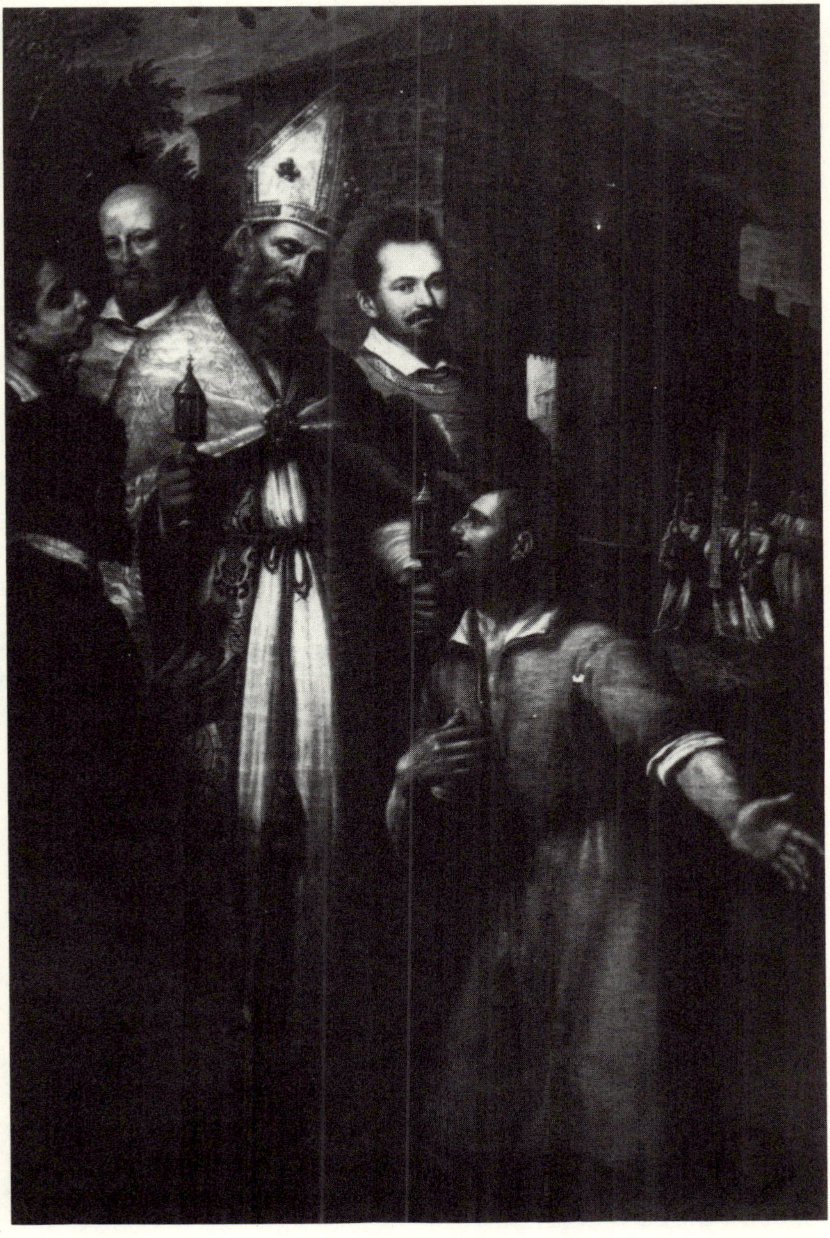

GLOSSARY

Abbreviations

Authorities cited

Identifications, alphabetically listed

Words, meanings, and ideas unfamiliar at present

Medicinals mentioned or used by Mercurialis

Proper names with brief biographical sketches, including

Paulus Aicardius
Cardinal Sirletus
Nicholas Culpeper and Robert James, who are frequently quoted herein

ABBREVIATIONS

acc	according to
adj	adjective
Ar	Arabic
AS	Anglo-Saxon
b	born
Bk	book, in *De Morbis Cutaneis*
ca	about
cap	with capital first letter
cf	compare
Ch	chapter
d	died
dim	diminutive
ed	educated (at)
Eng	English
esp	especially
fl	flourished
Fr	French
fr	from
Gr	Greek
Heb	Hebrew
L	Latin
lit	literally
med	medicine, medical, in medical usage
ML	Middle Latin
mod	modern, modern usage
NL	New Latin
obs	obsolete
OF	Old French
OHG	Old High German
p	page
part	participle
Per	Persian
pharm	pharmacologic, in pharmacology
Skr	Sanskrit
Sp	Spanish
sp	species

AUTHORITIES QUOTED IN GLOSSARY

Americana; The Encyclopedia Americana, New York, Chicago, and Washington, D.C., Americana Corporation (1955).

Baillon, M.E.: Dictionnaire de Botanique, Paris, Librairie Hachette et Cie, 1876-1892, 4 v.

Barton, Benjamin H., and Castle, Thomas: The British Flora Medica, London, Chatto and Windus, 1877.

Blase, Irene: see Foreword acknowledgment. Latinist.

Bowen, Lydia: see Foreword acknowledgment. Botanical librarian.

Britannica: Encyclopaedia Britannica, Encyclopaedia Britannica Inc., Chicago, London, Toronto, Wm. Benton (1956).

Butler, Dr. Roy F.: see Foreword acknowledgment. Baylor University classicist.

Celsus, Aurelius Cornelius: De medicina, with an Engl. transl. by W. G. Spencer, Cambridge, Mass., Harvard University Press; London, William Heinemann, Ltd., 1935-38. 3 v. (Half-title: The Loeb classical library. Latin authors.)

Coveney, Raymond M., Jr., Ph.D.: Minerologist, Professor of Geosciences, University of Missouri-Kansas City.

Culpeper, Nicholas, M.D.: Culpeper's Complete Herbal and English Physician, Enlarged, 1653, London, Richard Evans, 1815.

Dodoens, Remberg: A new Herball, or historie of plants . . . now first translated out of French . . . by Henry Lyte, London, 1595.

Dorland's Illustrated Medical Dictionary, Philadelphia and London, W. B. Saunders Co., 24th ed. 1965.

Eloy, N. F. J.: Dictionnaire Historique de la Medicine Ancienne et Moderne, Mons, 1778.

Garrison, Fielding H.: An Introduction to the History of Medicine, Philadelphia and London, W. B. Saunders Co., 4th ed. 1929.

Grieve, (Mrs.) M.: A Modern Herbal, New York, Hafner Co., 1931, 2 v.

Haseeb, Prof. Mansour Ali: see Foreword acknowledgment.

Husted, Jean: see Foreword acknowledgment. Dorland's Dictionary editor.

James, R.: Medical Dictionary, including Physic, Surgery, Anatomy, Chymistry, and Botany, in all their Branches relative to Medicine, together with a History of Drugs, an Account of their Various Preparations, Combinations, and Uses, and an Introductory Preface, Tracing the Progress of Physic, and explaining the Theories which have principally prevailed in all Ages of the World, London, printed for T. Osborne, sold by J. Roberts, 1745.

Lewis, Carlton T., and Short, Charles: A Latin Dictionary, founded on Andrews' Edition of Freund's Latin Dictionary, Oxford University Press, 1879.

Major, Ralph H., M.D.: A History of Medicine, Springfield, Ill., Charles C Thomas, 1954, 2 v. Univ. KS Prof. of Med.

Matthiole, Pietro Andrea: Commentarii in libros sex Pedacii Dioscoridis Anazarbei de medica materia, Venice, 1554, translated from Latin to French by M. Antoine du Pintet, Paris, 1680.

Mettler, Cecilia C., and Mettler, F. A.: History of Medicine . . . Philadelphia and Toronto, Blakiston, 1947.

Peters, Hermann: Pictorial History of Ancient Pharmacy, translated by William Netter, Chicago, G. P. Engelhard & Co., 1889.

Power, Henry, and Sedgwick, Leonard W.: The New Sydenham Society's Lexicon of Medicine and the Allied Sciences (Based on Mayne's Lexicon), London, The New Sydenham Society, 1881-99. 5 v.

Quincy, John: Dispensatory of the Royal College of Physicians in London. London, Pr. by W. Bowyer, for R. Knaplock (and others), 1721.

Sarton, George: Introduction to the History of Science, Baltimore, published for the Carnegie Institution of Washington by the Williams and Wilkins Co. (1927-48). 3 v. in 5.

Saunders, John B. de C. M., and O'Malley, Charles D.: Andreas Vesalius Bruxellensis: The Bloodletting Letter of 1539 . . . New York, Henry Schuman. (n.d.)

Skeat, Walter W.: Etymological Dictionary of the English Language, Oxford University Press, 3rd ed. impression of 1958.

Smith, William, editor: Dictionary of Greek and Roman Biography and Mythology. London, Murray, 1844-49. 3 v.

Turner, Daniel: De Morbis Cutaneis, A Treatise of Diseases Incident to the Skin . . . 3rd ed. London, R. & J. Bonwicke (and others), 1726.

Webster, 1918: Webster's New International Dictionary of the English Language, based on the International Dictionaries of 1890 and 1900, with a reference history of the World, W. T. Harris, Editor-in-Chief, F. S. Allen, General Editor, Springfield, Mass., G. and C. Merriam Co., 1918.

Webster, 1938: Webster's New International Dictionary of the English Language, 3rd ed. Unabridged, Wm. A. Neilson, Editor-in-Chief, Springfield, Mass., G. & C. Merriam Co., 1938. (Preface states, "In general, words which had become obsolete before 1500 have been omitted, but the whole vocabulary of Chaucer has been retained.")

Webster, 1962: Webster's New 20th Century Dictionary of the English Language, Unabridged, 2nd ed. Supervision of Editorial Staff by Jean L. McKechnie, Cleveland, World Publishing Co., 1962.

IDENTIFICATIONS

ABROTANUM (L): southernwood, an aromatic shrubby southern European wormwood, q.v., used in flavoring beer. "The leaves are reputed to have great success in destroying worms . . . The ancients commend it as good against all sorts of poisons, the bites and stings of venomous creatures, as likewise against obstructions of the liver, the jaundice, and to promote the menses," acc James.

ABSINTHIUM (L): wormwood, q.v.

ABSTERGENT (L abstergere, to wipe off): cleansing or purging, detersive, detergent, q.v.

ABSTERSIVE, noun: a medicine that is abstergent, q.v.

ACACIA (L fr Gr akakia, a thorny tree of Egypt): gum arabic, q.v., from trees of genus Acacia of the mimosa family, a nearly colorless gum, translucent, mucilaginous, emollient, demulcent.

ACETOSA (L acetum, vinegar, fr acere, to be sharp): the sour herb, sorrel, q.v. "The leaves are of great use against the scurvy," acc James.

ACHOR (Gr, scurf, dandruff, fr achyron, a heap of chaff): the scab or scald on the head, acc Lewis and Short. Three meanings are given by Dorland: an eruption of the face and scalp of infants, or an acuminate pustule. "An achor is an external sore of the head, full of little perforations, which discharge a humor much like ichor, whence the disease, or sore itself, is called an achor; Trallianus," acc James. See Book One, Chapter Nine. ?Atopic dermatitis, with or without secondary infection, fungal, bacterial or both.

ACROCHORDON: filiform mole or wart; a rounded excrescence on the skin with a slender base, regarding which Celsus stated that if it is cut out, it leaves no root and is not subject to grow again, acc Galen (Def. Medic.), said James, who, under verruca, wrote: "Sometimes a few capillaries putting out together do, after they have grown to a small length, enlarge themselves into a greater compass and make the pensile tumor we call acrochordon."

ACTION: Galen defined a disease as "such a preternatural disposition or affection of the parts of the body as primarily and of itself hinders their natural and proper action," acc James, who explained: "The actions, or functions, of the body are divided, by the writers of Institutes, into the vital, animal, and natural. The vital are such as are so necessary that the individual cannot subsist a few minutes without their exercise. Such is the motion of the heart and lungs; the secretion of spirits in the cerebellum, upon which the motion of the heart and lungs depends; and the circulation of the blood and spirits in their proper vessels. The natural actions are such as are necessary for the continuance of the animal, but not so immediately but that it can subsist a considerable time without them, as the digestion of the aliment and its conversion into blood. Under animal actions are comprehended those which constitute the senses of touch, taste, smell, vision, hearing, perception, imagination, memory, judgment, ratiocination, affections of the mind, and voluntary motion, without any or all of which an animal may live, but not very comfortably." See disease.

ACTUARIUS (Johannes the Actuarius, or scribe), fl ca 1250-1300, was a learned follower of Hippocrates and Galen and a court physician at Constantinople, the last of the Byzantine writers. His best known work was "On the Urines." He considered urine a filtrate of the blood, an excretion, valuable in diagnosis but not to the exclusion of other evidences of disease. He wrote also on the dependence of mental symptoms on organic causes, such as fatigue and intemperance, and prescribed diets, baths, and exercises for mental patients. (Major.)

ADARCE (Gr): a soft, porous, saltlike concretion on reeds and grass in marshy ground in Galatia, probably impure calcite and gypsum. It "is bred in moist and marshy places by drought, its color like that of the fine powder of the Assian stone (fr Aosos, a city of Troas), or sarcophagus, its substance lax and porous, much like the bastard sponge. It is a topic (agent applied topically) adapted to rub and scour the skin in a leprosy, sunburning, tetters, freckles, and such like blemishes. The adarce of Plotius is nothing but a concretion of stony particles of a white color, which one water at its meeting with another water incrusts grass, twigs, and other bodies floating by it," acc James. See pericalamitis. Sarcophagus (Gr sarx, flesh, and phagein, to eat) was a limestone, lapis Assius, used among the Greeks for coffins, which within a few weeks disintegrated the flesh of bodies deposited in it. (Webster, 1938.)

ADSTRINGENTS (fr L astringere, to draw tight): "Adstringents have such a particular conformation of their particles that they are able to draw and bind those about them to themselves, fastening them as if with little wedges, or tying them close with cords, upon which account they are most commonly of a cold nature," acc Turner.

AESCHINES, ca 389-314 B.C., an Athenian orator, was a political opponent of Demosthenes. He and Demosthenes were members of the first embassy to Philip (father of Alexander the Great), King of Macedonia, and was tried for treason for negotiations with Philip that were followed by Philip's conquest of Phocis. Mercurialis quoted his observation of white vitiligo in the inhabitants of Delos, an island in the Aegean. (Britannica.)

AETIUS (Aetios), 502-575, of Amida, on the Tigris, was the first Christian physician of note. His Tetrabiblion reflected Christian mysticism and pagan superstition, related magic formulae and incantations, and indicated his blind faith in the infallibility of Galen. He took much from Soranus, Oreibasios, Archiagenes, and Ruphos, as well as Galen. He gave good descriptions of diphtheria and poisons, produced a valuable treatise on ophthalmology, and was first to discuss camphor, cloves, and several other Eastern drugs later introduced in numbers by the Arabs. (Major.)

AGARIC (L agaricum, the larch or tinder fungus, fr Agaria, in ancient Sarmatia, that is, Poland and Russia west of the Volga): a gill fungus of genus Agaricus, or sp of Fomes that attack beech, elm, and various fruit trees; a pliant, feltlike material used to make punk; the dried fruit body of Fomes (Polyporus) officinalis that has been used internally to reduce perspiration. It is a slow purge with unpleasant features, acc James, who doubted the identification of the substances called agaric by the ancients and by his contemporaries.

AGARIC, PILLS OF: "Take of agarick 3 drams; our own blue orris roots, mastich, horehound, of each 1 dram; turbeth 5 drams; species hiera picra ½ ounce; colobynth and sarcocolla, of each 2 drams; myrrh 1 dram; and sape as much as is sufficient to make it into a mass according to art," acc Culpeper, who commented, "It was invented to cleanse the breast and lungs of flegm, it works pretty strongly. Half a dram at a time (keeping yourself warm) cannot well do you harm, unless your body be very weak."

AICARDIUS, PAULUS: was born at Albenga, an Italian port town on the Ligurian Sea about 50 miles from Monaco to the southwest and from Genoa to the northeast. He received his doctorate at Turin, about 100 miles north, and in 1570 moved to Padua, where his great erudition earned the esteem and friendship of the celebrated Jean-Vincent Pinelli (Italian patron of letters, 1535-1601), because of attachment to whom he several times refused more advantageous offers. Aicardius died in August of 1607. He published the treatise on Diseases of the Skin of Mercurialis and also wrote commentaries or remarks on many of the writers of antiquity, on Celsus among others; but all has been lost or scattered with the exception of his notes and variants on Julius Caesar, which Franz van Oudendorp (Dutch philologist, 1696-1761) adjoined to his edition of this author's works (Leyden, 1737). (Acc to Dictionaire des sciences medicale; A. Jourdan: Biographie medicale, C. L. F. Panckoucke, editeur, vol. 1, p. 77, Paris, 1820). Aicardius may be said to have been worshipful of Mercurialis, painstaking in his editorial work, somewhat tedious and repetitious, and understandably deficient in Greek as compared with the mentor.

ALBARA (fr L albus, white; albare, to make white; albarium, a kind of thin stucco for whitening walls): a skin disease characterized by pigment changes, practically synonymous with vitiligo, and with macular lesions. These may be white or dark; black albara was the lepra Graecorum. See Book Two, Chapters Two and Five.

ALBERTUS MAGNUS (Albert von Bollstädt), 1193-1280, b Lauingen in Swabia, canonized by Gregory XV in 1622, was the dominant figure of his time in Latin learning and natural science, the most prolific of writers, the most influential of teachers, the dean of scholars, the one man of learning of the twelfth and thirteenth centuries to be called "the Great." At 16 years of age he entered the Dominican order. He studied at Padua and Paris, became Bishop of Ratisbon but resigned to become a scholar, traveled much, spent considerable time at Cologne, where he organized a university in 1248, and wrote voluminously on theology, philosophy, chemistry, physics, botany, astronomy, geography, and zoology. An originator of the experimental school, he performed and recorded investigations of plants, animals, and chemicals. His works on natural sciences seem best and most original to modern readers, but he accepted many fantastic tales. Among his students were Roger Bacon, Thomas Aquinus, and Peter Hispanus, who became a pope. (Major.)

ALCONIUM (fr Ar al-koh'l, something subtle); alcohol.

ALCYON: acc James, "Alcyonium, bastard spunge, a sort of spungy plant which is found in the sea or upon the shore or rather a froth of the sea, which is hardened by the heat of the sun . . . What these bodies are has been a controverted point among the botanists and is not yet decided. Pliny writes they are the nests of some sort of bird . . . Dioscorides reckons five species: the hard bastard spunge resembles in some measure a sponge, but it is hard, heavy, and of a sour taste and disagreeable smell like a fish . . ." Other varieties, James said, are light and porous, smell like alga, or "in the form of little worms of a purple colour, sometimes white, sometimes yellow," or light, soft, and woolly, or resembling a mushroom, soft, rough within, and porous like pumice stone, without smell. James gave also, "Halcyonium, spuma maris, froth or foam of the sea, an oleous or bituminous substance found floating on the sea. It is much controverted whether this is the excrement, sperm, or milk of some sea animal, or a kind of zoophyte, or a juice of some sea plant, or something of a bituminous mineral exudation from the bottom of the sea, converted into foam by the agitation of the waves."

Spuma maris, acc Culpeper, "is hot and dry, helps scabs, itch, and leprosy, scald heads, etc.; it cleanses the skin, helps difficulty of urine, makes the teeth white being rubbed with it; the head being washed with it, it helps baldness, and trimly decks the head with hair."

Mod Alcyonaria is an order of Anthozoa with branched tentacles, of a shape presumably resembling the halcyon's nest. The halcyon, a kingfisher-like bird, was anciently thought to nest at sea at the time of the winter solstice in floating nests that calmed the waves. The sea fan and sea pen are familiar species. Alcyonarians are normally found only in deep water, usually attached to a foreign body. (Webster, 1962.)

ALEMBIC (L alembicum, fr Ar al-inbig, the still, fr Gr ambix, a cup, the cap of a still): an apparatus for distillation. Alembicate, to distill.

ALEXANDER OF TRALLES (an ancient town of Asia Minor, mod Guzel Hissar): 525-605, was a practitioner who traveled widely and settled at Rome. His father was a physician; his brothers, too, were distinguished. Anthemios, one of them, was the architect of St. Sophia at Constantinople. Alexander, a follower of Galen, was a Byzantine compiler, whose Practica showed some originality in descriptions of disease. Some of the prescriptions appear to be his own, notably those using burned substances. He was the greatest medical scholar between the time of Galen and the Renaissance. His Greek writings were translated into Latin, Syriac, Arabic, and Hebrew and had great influence during the Middle Ages. His books on pharmacy were required texts at the University of Paris five centuries later. His masterpiece was his Twelve Books on Medicine, in which he followed Hippocrates' and Galen's doctrine of the four humors, the composition of which determined the character of diseases, and accredited favorable effects on the patient of magical incantations and amulets, while quoting Aristotle, who said, when he disagreed with Galen, "I love Plato, but I also love the truth, so if a choice must be made, one must give preference to the truth." (Major.)

ALEXIPHARMIC (fr Gr alexein, to keep off, and pharmakon, poison): adj, counteracting poison, antidotal; noun, antidote.

ALHANDAL, or ALANDAHAL, TROCHES: "Take of coloquintida freed from the seeds and cut small, and rubbed with an ounce of oil of roses, then beaten into fine powder, 10 ounces; gum arabic, tragacanth, and bdellium, of each 6 drams. Steep the gums 3 or

4 days in a sufficient quantity of rose water till they be melted, then with the aforesaid pulp, and part of the said mussilage, let them be dried in the shadow, then beaten again, and with the rest of the mussilage, make it up again, dry them and keep them for use. They are too violent for a vulgar use," acc Culpeper. See colocynth, and troche.

ALICA (L): spelt, a kind of grain; or a drink prepared from it, acc Lewis and Short. James wrote: "A food much celebrated amongst the ancients, but the various accounts of it by different authors make somewhat uncertain what it was." He quoted Celsus as to its being a proper aliment in fevers, Aretaeus as to its being almost as good as ptisan, both being viscid, smooth, and pleasant to taste, and Dioscorides as to its being the double-grained sort of zea, more nourishing and binding than rice and helpful by topical application in lepra and roughness and scabbiness of the nails. Galen spoke of it as a kind of wheat. An invention of the Romans, acc Pliny, who distinguished it from the Gr chondrus (q.v.), saying it was made of zea pounded in a wooden mortar, not stone, to a coarse granular material. Alica, then, referred to the kind of meal rather than the kind of grain, acc James.

ALLIUM (L): garlic, q.v. The Allia are alliaceous plants of the lily family, including onion, garlic, and ascalonium (shallot).

ALKMAN (Alcmaeon), the poet, fl ca 670 B.C. about the time of Sappho, is recognized as the inventor of love songs, the founder of Doric lyric poetry. A Lydian of Sardis who came to Sparta as a slave, he lived with the family of Agesidas, by whom he was emancipated. His fondness for good living and taste for Asiatic sensuousness seemed out of place amid Spartan simplicity. His choral lyric voicing of the sentiments of a community was given in strophic arrangement, which came to be an essential of an ode. (Britannica.) Mercurialis mentioned him as one who died of pediculosis.

ALMOND (L amygdala): the small tree, Amygdalus communis, native to western Asia, resembling the peach in flowers but with dry fruits; or the drupaceous fruit, especially its ellipsoidal, slightly compressed, nutlike kernel. Cultivated from antiquity, the various kinds, bitter, sweet, hard-shell, soft-shell, and paper-shell, have developed from the single species.

Bitter almonds are grown mainly in the Mediterranean area and used in making flavoring extracts. Sweet almonds, eaten as nuts and used in cooking and confectionery, yield oil and are frequently ground to a paste or powder. Almond meal is used in cosmetics and perfumes. Almond cake is the residue after expressing oil. Almond milk, an emulsion of blanched almonds, acacia, sugar, and water, is used as a demulcent. Oil of bitter almonds owes its characteristic odor and flavor to benzaldehyde and contains prussic acid (hydrocyanic acid), which is removed when the oil is used for flavoring. Peach and apricot kernels yield a similar essential oil. (Webster, 1938.)

ALOE (L): a large genus of the lily family; leaves of A. vera the source of aloes, the purgative, tonic, and emmenagogue. "Aloes is no violent purge, is very friendly to the stomach, like wormwood. It purges bile and phlegm and may be taken every day after supper and would be a very fit purge for children were it not for its excess in bitterness, which children cannot endure," acc James.

ALTHAEA: malvaceous herbs including the marsh mallow, q.v.

ALUM (L alumen, from a stem signifying bitter): potassium aluminum sulfate, which is potassium alum; ammonium aluminum sulfate; or a mixture of these in large, clear, octahedral crystals, used as an astringent and styptic, internally as an emetic; also aluminum sulfate.

ALUM, BLACK (L alumen, alum; also an herb): the comfrey, a plant of genus Symphytum, Old World herbs of the borage family. S. officinalis, a kind of garlic formerly used to coagulate wounds, has 4 ovoid black nutlets, and the exterior of its roots is black: "It is said by Dioscorides to be so powerful to consolidate and knit together that if they be boiled with dissevered pieces of flesh in a pot it will join them together again," acc Culpeper, who stated that the comfrey is Consolida major; Consolida minor is the herb self-heal.

ALUMEN USTUM (L): burnt alum, which is alum dehydrated at 200° C and powdered, used as a caustic.

AMMI (L): A genus of umbelliferous plants of the parsley family, the Apiaceae, which includes bishop's weed, celery, carrot, parsnip, anise, and caraway. A. majus is the classic source of the contact photosensitizer methoxsalen, which has been used for many centuries in the treatment of depigmenting disorders. (Dorland.)

AMOMUM: "Dioscorides, particular in his account of it, but hard perplexed as to what it was," acc James, "described it as a small shrub that grows twisting its woody stem into the form of a bunch of grapes." James listed 3 plants known as amomum in 18th century use: bastard stone parsley, true amomum, and true night-shade. The true came mainly from the Philippine Islands and was a principal ingredient of Venice treacle as then prepared. Webster (1918) gave, "Any of various aromatic plants mentioned by the ancients but not certainly identified, obs; cap, a large genus of zinziberaceous plants of Asia, Africa, and Australia that yield aromatic seeds, the cardamoms and grains of paradise of commerce." Lydia Bowen wrote, "Stone parsley, Sison amomum, Umbelliferae, of Europe and Asia Minor is a possibility. Grieve (vol 2, p 612) says that the species has aromatic seeds. Dodoens (p 608) says that the stone parsley (Petropelinum macedonicum, which appears to be his species) is also called amomum by some ignorant apothecaries."

AMPELOLEUS: the "white vine" used by Mercurialis as a psilother was white bryony, q.v.

ANACARDINE CONFECTION: "a confection of anacardiums (cashew) which helps the memory, restores lost reason, removes a lethargy, and cures the gout, hemorrhoids, and those who are oppressed with melancholy or phlegm," acc James, whose formula contained emblic, myrobalan, pepper, ginger, honey of anacardium, castor, storax, cloves, camomile flowers, bayberries, cyperus, sugar, and honey.

ANASARCA (fr Gr ana, throughout, and sarkx, sarcos, flesh): dropsy, q.v., of the subcutaneous and intermuscular connective tissues, marked by soft, pale, inelastic swelling of the skin.

ANDROMACHUS THE ELDER, fl ca 50, of the school of Eristratos, a contemporary of Nero (37-68), lived after the time of Tiberius and Claudius and before Crito, who flourished under Trajan. He is known mainly through many descriptions of compound medicines, partly of his own invention, that have been transmitted by Galen. His best known he called "galene" (calm-procuring), also "eudeos" (serene) and "ilare" (cheerful), later known as theriaca, which he described in a Greek poem in elegaic verse, perhaps to make alterations of the formula easy to detect, Galen suggested. His theriaca superseded mithridate, q.v., although it was an imitation, acc James, differing mainly in that it contained viper flesh. "To this very day," said James, "the most considerable towns in Europe religiously follow the directions of Andromachus in their method of preparing it. This direction comprehends above sixty ingredients, the most part of which are aromatics except some common simples, gums, and inspissated juices, the most considerable of which is opium. But the vipers are the ingredients from which this medicine received the name theriaca, for the word therion among the Greeks imported all kinds of fierce animals, but more particularly such as were esteemed venomous." See hiera.

ANETHINE OIL (fr L anethum, dill): oil from dried ripe fruit of the dill, q.v., Anethum graveolens, used as carminative and stomachic; cf anise.

ANIMA (L): something breathing or blowing; wind, breath; breath of life, vital principle, life, soul. Prima materia, primary matter, has the potentiality of being molded by anima, the vital force; things are form-matter (anima-materia) compounds. See materia.

ANISE (L anisum, fr Ar anisun): a plant of the carrot family, Pimpinella anisum, native of Egypt, cultivated for its fragrant seeds. Anise seed, aniseed; see Ammi, and anethine oil.

ANTIDOTE (L antidotum, Gr antidoton fr anti, against, and didonai, to give): a remedy against a poison. See dose, mithridate, and theriac.

APERIENTS (fr L aperire, to uncover, open): medicines for opening, loosening, flushing, which "by their slender and sharp pointed particles are able to insinuate themselves deeply into the body, where breaking in sunder the more crass and terrene (particles) they enter their pores and open the obstructed passages; and of such there are both hot and cold. On the other side, such as thicken and incrassate, work their effect by their more gross and ramous parts, mixing with and entangling others that are more moist and liquid and uniting or joining themselves therewith, encrease the consistence of the same, these are generally cold in quality," acc Turner.

APHRONITER: flowers, q.v., of saltpeter, q.v.

APIUM (L): parsley; smallage, or wild celery, acc James. Cap, a genus of apiaceous herbs native to southern Europe and mountainous tropical regions; A. graveolens, garden celery. See Ammi.

APOLLONIUS ("Biblias," the bookworm) of Kitium, fl ca 160 B.C., of the Empiric School, wrote a commentary on the Hippocratic treatise on dislocations, remarkably illustrated by Niketas (900), whose surgical collection, purchased in 1495 for Lorenzo de Medici, is in the Laurentian Library at Florence. (Garrison.)

APPENDAGE (fr L ad-pendere, hang to): something appended to, an appurtenance. Mod, appendages of the skin are hairs, nails, sweat glands, oil glands, and apocrine glands.

APPONENSIS (Peter of Abano), ca 1250-1316, was the first medical professor to give Padua a wide reputation. After preliminary study in Greece and Constantinople, he moved to Paris, studied philosophy, mathematics, and medicine, became known as "the Great Lombard," and returned to Padua to teach. His rationalistic philosophy made him suspect of being a follower of Averroes, and his knowledge of alchemy and astrology made him suspect as a magician. He was tried twice by the Inquisition, died during the second trial, was later adjudged guilty. Lacking his bones, they burned him publicly in effigy. Best known were his works on poisons and his "Conciliation," an effort to reconcile conflicts of Arabic with Greek medicine and disputes on astronomy, mathematics, and geography. He gave considerable credence to the importance of astrology in treating disease. (Major.) See p. xxxix.

APPULEIUS, ca 400, was author of a herbarium popular for centuries, of which the material was borrowed largely from Pliny and Dioscorides. Its relationship is unclear to the herbarium of "Pseudo-Appuleius Platonicus," printed in Rome in 1480 from a medieval manuscript that summarized medical knowledge and consisted of a hodgepodge of gleanings from Greek and Latin authors. (Garrison; Major.)

ARCHIGENES (Archiagenes of Apamea in Asia Minor) fl ca 100, was a contemporary of Celsus and practiced in Rome during the time of Trajan (53-117). Son of a renowned physician, he was a man of great learning who shed luster on the Eclectic School and wrote many medical books on the pulse, fevers, surgery, drugs, and therapeutics that were quoted respectfully by Galen. Aretaios and Aetios copied from him freely without acknowledging their indebtedness, acc Major.

ARISTOTLE, 384-322 B.C., son of a physician, Plato's most famous pupil, was one of the greatest philosophers and scientists. He wrote on logic, geometry, astronomy, and mechanics, carried out investigations in botany, zoology, anatomy, and physiology, stated clearly some fundamental problems of biology regarding sex, heredity, nutrition, growth, and adaptation, proposed a theory of evolution, and devised the first scientific classification of animals. He studied the uterus of various animals and the embryology of the chick. He believed the heart to be the seat of intelligence and thought arteries contain air. (Major.)

ARRIANUS (FLAVIUS ARRIAN), ca 100-170, Greek historian, of Nicomedia in Bithynia, lived during the reigns of Hadrian and Marcus Aurelius. Hadrian made him governor of Cappadocia, the only instance prior to the third century when a Greek was given a major Roman command. He was a pupil and friend of Epictetus, and published his lectures on the history of Alexander the Great, the best source extant on the subject. (Britannica.)

ARSENIC: see realgar.

ASCALONIUM (fr L ascalonius, of Ascalon, a seacoast town in southern Palestine): the shallot, Allium ascalonicum, of the lily family, an onionlike plant having small, clustered bulbs, used for flavoring; leek, scallion, eschalot. Allium sativum is garlic, q.v.

ASPLENIUM (NL fr L asplenum, spleenwort, fr Gr a-, euphonic, and splenon, the spleen): polypodiaceous ferns, the spleenworts, also known as miltwaste, which include the familiar maidenhair fern. "A small plant, three or four inches long," acc James, "consisting of leaves which spring from a fibrous root, the leaves greenish on the upper side and brownish and full of dusty seed underneath, generally crumpled or folded inward, in shape something like the insect scolopendra, from which it takes one of its names" (see scolopendrium). Supposedly good in diseases of the spleen, "it also opens obstructions of the liver, helps the jaundice, and is very good for the rickets in children."

ATHENAEUS, fl ca 50, from Attalia in Asia, practiced in Rome during the reigns of Claudius and Nero. He wrote a treatise of 30 books on medicine, only a few fragments of which have been preserved. He was the founder of the Pneumatists, who were not rigid in dogma but chose what they thought best of the Dogmatists, Empiricists, and Methodists and hence came to be known as the Eclectics. It was their view that pneuma, the vital principle that controls the body, is drawn in from the air via respiration and the skin pores and distributed by the blood vessels. Health represents a normal state of the pneuma; disease, an improper mixture or "dyscrasis" of the humors, which causes a disturbance of the pneuma. (Major.)

ASTRAMENTUM SUTORIUM (L, lit shoemaker's black): vitriol, q.v., acc James; presumably an impure mixture of salts and oxides of iron.

ATTENUANTS (fr L attenuare, to make thin, less viscid; L tenuis, thin): thinning, diluting medicines, which "are such as by their acute parts divide and cut in sunder the viscid or tough humors, breaking them into particles smaller and more fine," acc Turner.

ATTENUATE: to effect the action of an attenuant, q.v.

ATTRAHENT (fr L attrahere, ad- and trahere, to draw to): a medicine which by irritation attracts action to the parts to which it is applied. A sinapism, q.v.; medicines "such as draw forth the humors (to which belong the pyroticks, burning and blistering medicines) exert their force and bring about their effects by their great heat and subtilty of parts, opening the pores, attenuating the humors, and forcing them from their receptacles. Some of them only swell and inflame the part, whilst others exciting great quantity of the serous latex to ouze forth off the glandules, and impelling the same against the cuticle, whose density confining them and keeping them in, they raise the same into a bladder; or else when of a more intense degree of heat, like that of fire, they burn the part into a crust or eschar," acc Turner.

AVENZOAR (Ibn Zuhr), ca 1091-1162, b Sevilla of a distinguished Spanish family and son of a prominent physician, was the greatest clinician of the Western Caliphate, a clear thinker little enamored of metaphysical subtleties, a fact which explains his lack of enthusiasm for Avicenna's Canon, the pages of which Avenzoar's father used for scratch paper. He was a vigorous opponent of astrology and mysticism. His influence in Europe was great. In his chief work, a treatise on clinical medicine, he emphasized the view that experience, not speculation, should guide the physician. He gave one of the earliest descriptions of the itch mite: "There move about sometimes in the body under the surface of the skin very small lice, and when the skin is scratched there come out living animals so very small that they can scarcely be seen." (Major.)

AVERROES (Ibn Ruschd), 1126-1198, b Cordoba of a family distinguished in law, studied philosophy, law, and medicine, with particular emphasis on the first. In his attempt to harmonize faith and reason, he evolved views that attracted many devoted followers and for several hundred years influenced religious thought. They resembled those of St. Thomas, but his doctrine that the soul of man is absorbed into universal nature at death was contrary to the teachings of Muslims and Christians, by both of whom he was considered impious. Soon after 1195, when the Muslim orthodox reaction flamed, he was banished, along with many other distinguished scholars. His General Rules of Medicine, much influenced by Aristotle, was a resumé of the medical sciences in seven books estimated by some as "a work written in the library rather than at the bedside." (Major.)

AVICENNA (Ibn Sina), 980-1037, b Ashena, Persia, became eminent as a physician, philosopher, scientist, statesman, and poet, his genius comparable with that of Leonardo and Goethe. At 10 years of age he was able to recite the Koran by heart. At 18 as a physician he was summoned to treat a prince, and at 21 he had compiled an encyclopedia of all sciences but mathematics. His poetry in Persian has been highly praised by literary critics. His cool intellectual outlook has been compared with that of

Averroes. His essay on the origin of mountains made him known as "the father of geology." His hundred or more books include his Canon, a huge unwieldy storehouse of learning intended to codify the whole of the medical knowledge of his time and to align the facts with the views of Galen and Aristotle, attempting to follow exact rules of logic. Called "the most famous medical textbook ever written," it was required reading at the University of Vienna 500 years after publication. It was weak in anatomy, which, denied by Islam to its scientists, was copied from Galen. Avicenna substituted the cautery for the knife where possible. His works intimated that surgery is an inferior art, a separate branch of medicine. He was first to describe the preparation and properties of sulfuric acid and alcohol, and he noted the sweet taste of the urine in diabetes. (Major.)

BALM OF GILEAD: a small evergreen tree, Commiphora meccanensis, of Africa and Asia, provides the leaves which when bruised yield a strong aromatic odor. Balsam from this plant is the commercial balm known also as balsam of Mecca, valued as an unguent and cosmetic by the Turks. See calamint.

BARBERRY (L berberis fr Ar barbaris): shrub of genus Berberis; red berries, used in preserves, have been used in treatment of fluxes and fevers.

BDELLIUM (L fr Gr bdellion fr Heb bedholah): a gum resin from various balsameaceous trees of genus Balsamea, resembling myrrh; mentioned in Bible, Gen ii, 12, and Num xi, 7, acc Webster (1938).

BETONY (L betonica): labiate plants including Eurasian herb Betonica officinalis, wood betony, an obs medicinal, the tops astringent and aromatic, the root emetic and cathartic; also the lousewort, stinking hellebore, or stavesacre, q.v.

BISHOP'S WEED: see Ammi.

BITTER ALMONDS: see almonds.

BITTERS: a pharmacologic liquor containing extracts of bitter herbs, leaves, or roots, used as a mild tonic or stimulant of appetite and digestion; aromatic b. contain aromatic oils, astringent b. contain tannin, simple b. practically free of aromatic oils and tannin, acc Webster (1938).

BLOOD (L sanguis): the humor, q.v., originating in the stomach, its dominant element air, dominant qualities hot and moist, the associated complexion (q.v.) sanguine, i.e. sturdy, ruddy, and cheerful; mod adj sanguine, confident, optimistic.

BOLUS (L): lit a rounded mass; med a large pill.

BORAGE (L borago, ? fr Ar abu-rashsh, father of sprinkling, source of sweat, related to med use): a small genus of Boraginaceae that are perennial herbs native to Mediterranean region; a European salad herb used as a demulcent and diaphoretic; "hot and moist in the first degree (mildly), cheers the heart, helps drooping spirits, acc to Dioscorides," acc Culpeper. Borage family includes bugloss, q.v.

BOTHOR (Ar butur, "t" sounded like Eng "th"; singular, batr): papulopustular lesions, translated "nodules" by Paul Richter (Archiv. f. Dermat. u. Syth. 112: 849, 1912); see Haly Abbas. Mercurialis used the word once in reference to Avicenna's differential diagnosis of scabies.

BRASSICA (L, cabbago): large genus of European, Asiatic, and African plants that include cauliflower, kale, Brussels sprouts, rape, turnip, rutabaga, and black mustard.

BROAD-BEAN, or horse-bean (L faba, fr Skr fag-va, to share food, Gr Phagein, to eat; cf Eng phage): a bean of family Fabaceae, formerly classed with Leguminosae, with fruit in pods, including the vetches.

BRODIUM (NL): "A pharmaceutical term signifying the same as jusculum" (fr L ius, iuris, broth; dim, presumably a thin broth; Eng broth fr AS, akin to OHG brod, a thin simple soup; of Gr oyron, L urina, Eng urine); "The liquor in which some medicine is preserved or with which something else is diluted," acc James.

BRYONY (L brionia): perennial, Old World, herbaceous, tendril-bearing vines of cucumber family. White bryony had virtue as a purgative and as a psilother; see ampeloleuce. "The root with bitter vetches, earth of Chios, and fenugreek absterges and clears the skin from wrinkles, sunburns, freckles, and black marks," acc James, quoting Dioscorides. Black bryony had much the same properties as white, but was less efficacious and was not a purge; it possessed violent properties and possibly was poisonous, not to be used in place of white bryony, James said.

BUCKTHORN: a shrub or tree of genus Rhamnus. The bark of cascara buckthorn, called chittem bark, is the source of the laxative, cascara. Cascara sagrada (Sp, sacred bark) comes from California buckthorn, Rhamnus purshiana, the bear-wood or bearberry.

BUGLOSS (L buglossa): various plants, including those of genus Anchusa, oxtongue, the source of alkanet, a red coloring used for tinctures, pomades, and beverages. Lycopsis arvensis, the wild bugloss, is of a genus of bristly herbs of the borage family, q.v.

BYZANTINE SYRUP: see syrup.

CACOCHYMIA (Gr kako, bad, and chymos, juice): a vitiated state of the humors or juices, esp of the blood. Eng chemistry is fr alchemy, fr ML alchimia, fr Ar al-kimiya, probably fr Gr chymos, juice, acc Webster (1938). See disease.

CALAMINE: see spodium, and Cimolian earth. ZnO with a little Fe_2O_3. (Coveney.)

CALAMINT: a mint of genus Calamintha, synonymous with Clinopodium, a large genus of menthaceous herbs or undershrubs of north temperate zone, including sp of basil, balm, and calamint.

CALVITIES (fr L calvus, bald; L calvarium, bare skull; L calva, scalp without hair): baldness. See Book One, Chapter Five.

CAMOMILE (L chamomilla, earth apple, fr odor of flowers): plant of genus Anthemis or related genera; dried flower heads used in aromatic bitters; camomile tea, an old household remedy.

CANNA (L): Rootstock of edible canna yields a kind of arrowroot.

CANTHARIDES (plural of L cantharis, fr Gr, a kind of beetle): A medicinal made from the Spanish fly, Lytta (Cantharis) vesicatoria; or the impure vesicant from this insect, a powerful rubefacient (q.v.) and, internally, a dangerous nephrotoxic substance alleged to be aphrodisiac. Cantharidin, the main active ingredient, is a lactone of cantharidic acid, $C_{10}H_{12}O_4$.

CAPILLUS (L): a hair of the scalp as distinguished from hair of other parts of the body, e.g. pilus, q.v.

CARMINATIVE (fr L carminare, to card, hence to cleanse): an agent for expelling wind, relieving colic.

CARTHAMUS (NL, fr Ar quirtim, safflower): Carthamus tinctorius, of a small genus of Eurasian herbs of the thistle family. The large, orange flowers were the source of "bastard saffron," much used in dyeing silk. The seeds were medicinal, "accounted a pretty strong cathartic," acc James, "evacuating phlegm both upwards and downwards, but prejudicial to the stomach."

CARYOPHYLLUS: the pinks and carnations; oil of, oil of cloves.

CASCARA: see buckthorn.

CASSIA (L): herbs, shrubs, and trees native of warm regions, the caesalpiniaceous herbs, the leaves of some species yielding senna; or pods of the pudding-pipe tree, C. fistula, the source of a sweet pulp, cassia pulp, which is a mild laxative. Cf tamarind.

CASSIUS (Cassius Felix), fl 130, wrote a book in Greek, a Latin translation of which appeared some three centuries later. He was one of the last representatives of Roman medicine. (Major.)

CASTOR (L, beaver): a bitter, orange-brown substance of strong, penetrating odor, found in two glandular sacs between the anus and external genitals of the beaver, used in obs medicine as a stimulant and antispasmodic, and by perfumers. Bean-size conglomerates of this sebaceous odorous substance may be dropped by a fleeing animal; these were mistaken for its testicles by the Egyptians, who were said by Horapollus, acc Faber's Lexicon, to paint a beaver when they intended to represent a man who castrates himself, a vulgar error, Dioscorides recognized, because the testicles in fact lie concealed, adherent to the spina dorsi, acc James. Castor was imported from Poland, Russia, and the East and West Indies. That of Canada was the worst, James said, "because it is almost void of smell, and that which it diffuses is ungrateful." For perhaps 2500 years it was used internally and externally for the most diverse conditions, particularly "for provoking the menses and in tremors, convulsions, and all diseases of the nerves." Topically it was a mild rubefacient, "to be rubbed into those parts which stand in need of a greater degree of heat."

CATAPLASM (fr Gr kataplassein, to mold down over, to spread over): a poultice.

CATAPOTION (Gr kata-, down, downward, in accordance with, against, completely, plus L potio, draft, dose, drug): a pill.

CAUSATION: Aristotle gave four kinds of causes in the processes of changing or becoming. The formal cause is the form or conception of that which is to be, as it exists ideally, either in the essential nature of things themselves or in the mind, e.g. the plan of a house in the mind of a builder. The material cause is that which is to be wrought to this form, e.g. the bricks and timber for the construction of the house. The efficient or moving cause is analogous to the labor expended in the building of the house. The final cause is that which is the end or object of the process, e.g. the finished house. (Webster, 1938.) Re causes of diseases, see disease.

CEDRIA (L): resin from the cedar tree; the tears or pitch from the tree, acc James, distinguished from that which is boiled or prepared from the juice of the cedar tree and known as cedrium.

CELERY (fr Gr selino, parsley): a European herbaceous plant, Apium graveolens, q.v.

CELSUS, AURELIUS CORNELIUS, ca 25 B.C.-50, was considered by Pliny a man of letters rather than of medicine. His De Medicina, neglected by contemporaries, was one of the first medical books to be printed (1478). It went through many editions, a fact due in part to the precision and purity of Celsus' literary style (Garrison). Of its eight books, the sixth concerned the skin and venereal diseases, as well as those of the eye, ear, nose, throat, and mouth, and described various dermatoses, ulcerations, condylomata, hemorrhoids, and cancer of the penis. His book on surgery included a description of an operation for carcinoma of the lower lip. See the translation by W. G. Spencer, Cambridge, Mass., Harvard University Press, 1935-1938. I must paraphrase an admonition Celsus wrote for medical students in an opening paragraph on surgery: "Do not be dismayed by the outcries of the patient since what you are doing is for his own good."

CERIA (fr L cera, beeswax): favus; see Book One, Chapter Nine.

CHALCANTHITE (fr Gr, flowers of bronze): blue vitriol, copper sulfate; or vitriol inexplicitly, confusing the blue and the green, the former a caustic metallic poison, the latter being ferrous sulfate, medicinally valuable. "The blue, or Roman, vitriol, known also as celestial stone and chalcalthum of Cypres, is constipating, provokes vomiting, expels worms, and is much commended for scabies and ulcers due to lues venerea," acc James, who described also green vitriol, copperas, and white vitriol, from Germany, presumably alum, and mentioned a red vitriol but said he had been unable to learn what it is—mercuric sulfide? Re toxicity see p. xxxiv.

CHALYBEATE (fr Gr Chalybes, the ancient people of Pontus, who were celebrated for working with iron and steel): impregnated with iron salts.

CHEMISTRY: see cacochimia.

CHICK-PEA (L cicer): Asiatic herb bearing short pods with one or two seeds resembling peas in flavor, important as an article of diet in southern Europe and India.

CHICORY (L cichoreum): a common European perennial plant cultivated as a salad herb and for its roots, which are roasted to mix with coffee; see lactuca. Several species were distinguished by James, including endive and wild and garden succory.

CHOLCODEUM: appearing once, the word is presumably a synonym of "creative," with a meaning resembling "concoctive." It has not been identified by consultants competent in Latin, Greek, and Arabic.

CHOLER (Gr chole, bile): the humor, yellow bile, originating in the heart, dominant element fire, dominant quality hot and dry, the associated complexion choleric, which now means easily moved to anger, hot tempered.

CHONDRUS (L): same as alica, q.v. Acc James, "It signifies also any grumous concretion, as of mastic or frankincense, and is, besides, the Gr word for a cartilage." In botany, Chondrus is a kind of red algae with coarse, branching fronds, including carrageen, a dark purple, cartilaginous seaweed from the coasts of northern Europe and North America, which when dried and bleached is the commercial Irish moss, acc Webster (1918).

CIMOLIA, CIMOLIAN EARTH (fr Gr island, Kimolos, in the Aegean Sea): a grayish or reddish, chalky aluminum silicate resembling calamine, identified by James as tobacco-pipe clay when white, fuller's earth when reddish, useful topically and as a cleanser when saponaceous. Soapstone, which is massive talc or steatite, is an acid metasilicate of magnesium, which sepiolite, or meerschaum, resembles chemically. Talcum and argillum (clay) were distinguished by the ancients, "The clays used in medicine being known in the shops by the name of terrae, or earths," acc James, who listed 15 of them, including terra Cimolia (alba and purpurascens) and t. Eretria, which Mercurialis used.

CITRON (L citrus, whence Gr kitron): originally the fruit of the lime and the lemon; mod the fruit of the tree, Citrus medica, the tree itself,or the preserved rind of the fruit, used in fruitcake, puddings, etc. See citrus.

CITRONWOOD: see sandarac.

CITRUS (L): the originally tropical Asian tree, the citron. Citron, a small genus of trees and shrubs, often thorny, of the rue family, is widely cultivated for citrus fruits: C. medica, the citron; C. limonia, the lemon; C. aurantifolia, the lime; C. sinensis, the orange; C. aurantiam, the bitter orange.

CLAUDIANUS, "friend of Galen" (b 130), who cured calvities with pericalamitis (adarce): ? Claudius Agathinus of Sparta, prominent Pneumatist, who was a pupil of Athenaeus of Attilia, who founded the Pneumatic school, and a teacher of Archigenes.

CLAY (L terra): see cimolia.

CLOVES: see caryophyllus.

COCHIA: certain officinal pills, the prescription originally Arabic. Acc James the "greater pill cochiae" contained hiera picra, troches of alhandal, diagrydium, turpeth, and syrup of buckthorn (cascara), a formula taken from Rhazes. The "lesser pill" contained aloes, scammony, colocynth, syrup of buckthorn, and oil of cloves. "A grain or two of opium is generally mixed with it to make its operation milder." "Pill cochiae with hellebore" contained the ingredients of the lesser pill, plus powder of black hellebore and syrup of stoechas, "an admirable cathartic . . . In a dose of gr xv to gr xxx its first use will sometimes vomit, but after a few repetitions it takes more downwards."

COLD SEEDS: see seeds.

COLOCYNTH (L colocynthis, fr Gr kolokynthis): Mediterranean and African herbaceous vine allied to watermelon, called also coloquintida, the bitter apple, cucumber, or gourd. From the dried pulp of unripe but full-grown fruit of Citrullus colocynthus is prepared a powerful cathartic, "a drug of great esteem in Medicine for many ages," said James, "but rough and violent." In the old Arabian preparation, trochischi alhandal, it was corrected with gummy and mucilaginous bodies, but "It is so smart a purger as not to be safe but to athletic constitutions."

COLOQUINTIDA: colocynth.

COLUMELLA, LUCIUS IUNIUS MODERATUS, of Gades, fl ca 50, a contemporary of Seneca, was a writer on agriculture. His extant works, which consist in the main of his De Arboribus and the twelve books of his De Re Rustica, one of which is in dactylic hexameter in imitation of Virgil, treat of the cultivation of all kinds of corn and garden vegetables, trees, flowers, the vine, and the olive and other fruits and of the rearing of cattle, birds, fishes, and bees. (Britannica.)

COMPLEXION (L complexio, combination, fr complector, twine around, embrace): the combination or properties of the humors and the qualities, hot, cold, moist, and dry, that determine the nature of the individual: the body constitution or habit; see constitution, elements, habitus, temperament.

CONCOCT (L concoquere, to cook together, digest, mature): to prepare, perfect, refine chemically by heat; to digest; to compose, devise, make. See digestion.

CONCOCTION: that which is concocted, i.e. prepared by heating together. Views of Aristotle on generation of lice by concoction are discussed in Book One, Chapter Seven, on Pediculosis.

CONDENSING MEDICINES: "by their coldness, restrain their motion so that falling as it were together they are more closely joined and connected to each other," acc Turner.

CONFECTION: a composition of drugs that included sugar, syrup, or honey to make a soft, palatable solid; an electuary.

CONFECTION OF HAMECH: a complex formula named after an

Arabian physician (Hamech was the name of the father of Mesuë Junior, who died 1015 A.D.) "a very ancient Arabian composition and first prescribed by Mesuë, so nauseous as seldom to be prescribed but in clysters, and not often neither in that manner . . . Difficult to keep because of (its) readiness to ferment," acc Quincy. Culpeper's formula contained myrobalan, chebula, colocynth, polypody, wormwood, thyme, anise, fennel, agaric, senna, rhubarb, fumitory, prune pulp, cinnamon, ginger, sugar and honey, and other things, a "receipt chiefly appropriate as a purge for melancholy and salt flegm, and diseases thence arising, as scabs, itch, leprosies, cancers, infirmities of the skin; it purges and adjusts humors, is good against madness, melancholy, forgetfulness, vertigo. It purges very violently and is not safe given alone. I would advise the unskillful not to meddle with it inwardly."

CONSTITUTION (L constitutio, Gr katastasis): physical organization; complexion, q.v.; habitus, q.v.

COOT: see phalacrocorax.

COPPER GREEN: "mineral green," a carbonate of copper; malachite.

COPPERAS (fr L cuperosa, ? for aqua cuprosa, copper water): crystallized ferrous sulfate, green vitriol, q.v.

CORIANDER (fr Gr koris, bedbug, because of its fetid odor): Old World herb of carrot family, its aromatic fruits, or "seeds," were used as stomachic and carminative and for seasoning.

CORNARIUS, JANUS, edited the Basel Opera Omnia of Hippocrates, printed by Froben (1538) and prized for its textual and critical accuracy. (Garrison.)

CORRECT (L, past part of corrigere, to make straight): to set straight, remove faults; to counteract through opposite qualities, to prevent or remove the effect, or neutralize the ill effect, of a medicine; to mollify excessive actions of a medicine.

CORRECTIVE: a medicinal agent to correct.

CORRUPT (L corrumpo, spoil, mar, make worse): spoiled, damaged, defective, tainted, vitiated, morbid, bad, depraved, incorrect, altered from sound to putrid state.

CORRUPTION: that which is corrupt; decay, decomposition; pus.

CRITO (Titus Statilius Crito), ca 100, was a Gr physician who practiced at the court of Trajan. Galen quoted much of his work on cosmetics and drugs.

CROCUS: see saffron; cf carthamus.

CRUST (L crusta): mod, an accumulation of dried serum and pus; a scab, q.v.

CTESIAS, of Cnidos, ca 400 B.C., a contemporary of Hippocrates, ed Alexandria, was a physician in the army of Cyrus, king of Persia. He visited India and wrote a treatise on Indian medicine, noting that the Indians were more skilled at treating snake bite than the Greeks. His writings include works on rivers, medicinal plants, and the history of Persia and Assyria. (Major.)

CULPEPER, NICHOLAS, 1616-1654, "set up as a physician and astrologer and soon achieved great fame and a large practice," Major wrote (p. 546); "He had studied at Cambridge and was at one time apprenticed to an apothecary in Bishopsgate. He was a great student and translated into English Galen's Ars parva, Rivier's work, Riolan's and Vesling's anatomies, and Sennert's Practice, and he edited an English edition of Glisson's De rachitide. His crowning offense in the eyes of his colleagues was his English translation of the London Pharmacopoeia, which, by custom and tradition, was in Latin. This translation, which his enemies asserted had been 'done very filthily into English,' was published in 1649. Culpeper's Herbal, published in 1653, went through many editions and was especially popular in the North American colonies. Culpeper at best was a quack and lacked scientific training, but he did popularize medical knowledge." Garrison, whose list (p 274) of the queer ingredients of the various editions of the London Pharmacopoeia is fascinating, noted that a reprint (1708) of Culpeper's Herbal appears to have been the first medical book published in the American colonies, and said of him: "While Culpeper indulged in a vast amount of scurrilous raillery at the expense of the London Pharmacopoeias of 1618 and 1650, except for his herb-lore he was himself only the credulous astrologer described by Nedham as a 'frowsy-headed coxcomb who had gallimawfried the Apothecaries' Book into nonsense in his aim to monopolize to himself all the knavery and cozenage that ever an apothecary's shop was capable of.'"

I have quoted Culpeper extensively because his material is colorful, provocative, irreverent of stuffed-shirt authorities, informative, and representative of the views of the times whether or not his more dignified counterparts chose to affect Latin. They all used about the same drugs with about the same rationale. He expressed his views honestly and without bias, when he said of hiera logadii he'd be reluctant to use it himself, even as a clyster.

CUMIN (L cuminum): apiaceous plant native to Egypt and Syria. The seeds, bitter, warm, and aromatic, are used as caraway seeds are.

CUP: verb, to apply cupping glass for bleeding a patient.

CUPPING GLASS (L cucurbitula, fr cucurbita, gourd, cup): a cup for drawing blood to the surface by applying suction to an area of the skin. Hippocrates used the device, with or without preliminary scarification (q.v.), respectively known as wet, or sanguineous, and dry cupping, acc James. "Before the application of the glass, a lighted candle, or fire, is to be conveyed into it that the air being expelled by the heat, the glass may immediately be adapted to, and impressed upon, the body till it firmly adheres with a strong attraction."

CUTTLEBONE: the calcarious internal shell of the cuttlefish, a ten-armed marine cephalopod. The structure distinguishes cuttlefish from squid and octopus. The bone, calcarious, was given "as a good diurectic. Others make a powder of it for cleaning the teeth. It dries and absterges, cures spots, freckles, and the humid itch, is good for the eyes, removes swellings in the gums, stops a gonorrhea, expels a stone, and provokes urine," acc James. See sepia.

CYATHUS (Gr kyathos, fr chyein, to pour out): a common measuring ladle of both liquid and dry substances, 1/12th of a sextarius, or 1 ounce, for taking one draught of liquor from a bowl, acc James. The several vessels that contained respectively 2, 3, 4, 5, and 6 cyathi, for example, were called the sextans, quadrans, triens, quinquax, and semis. A Roman at an entertainment might drink a cyathus of wine for each letter spelling the name of his patron, along with 9 for the Muses and 3 for the Graces. Mercurialis mentioned the measure once.

CUPERUS (L cyperum): sedge, plants resembling grasses but with solid stems; species include forage plants, basket and mat-weaving material, chufa with its edible roots, and papyrus, q.v. James listed several, attributing to them medicinal properties such as heating, drying, expelling wind, strengthening the bowels, and helping giddiness. Hippocrates recommended cyperus for diseases of the uterus.

DECOCTION (fr L decoctus, fr decoquere, to boil down): something prepared, digested, or extracted by hot or boiling water; or prepared by the heat of the stomach.

DEFLUVIUM (fr L defluo, flow, slip, fall down): falling of the hair; see Book One, Chapter Three.

DELPHINIUM: larkspur; see staphisagria.

DERMA (Gr): mod, the corium, the part of the skin beneath the epidermis, external to the fatty layer. It becomes leather when a hide is tanned. Mercurialis did not use the word; see epidermis.

DETERGENTS (fr L detergere, to rub or wipe off): cleansing agents or solvents; cleansing medicines, which "may be said to operate by their hard, rough, and pointed particles, scouring and cleansing away the filth sticking in the passages, against which they happen to be impelled, or upon which they fasten," acc Turner.

DEW (L, ros): James wrote, "If in a long continued summer's drought, the surface of the earth comes to be greatly parched with the heat of the sun, not only water, but also other less volatile substances, of an unctuous and saline nature, will thus be raised to some height into the atmosphere, tho invisibly, so long as such exhalations are agitated by the sun's heat, which coming to lessen towards the evening, the air soon grows cooler; while at the same time, the earth retaining the heat much longer than the air, still continues to breathe out hot exhalations, whence arises a white, dense, visible vapour, hotter below than above, and this vapor appears, therefore, first in low watery places, thence gradually diffuses itself so as in the night to cover the surface of the earth with a mist, which is dissipated by the rising sun. This moisture, called by the name of Dew, is a very compound substance, nor can be asserted anything that will hold universally true of its peculiar nature. It must needs be a chaos, as it is a collection of all sorts of volatile particles, promiscuously jumbled together by the heat of the sun, acting upon the earth; it must also be different in different parts of the earth, according as different kinds of particles lodge therein. Thus in large tracts of gravelly or heath ground, which lie high and dry, it will be small in quantity, and almost totally aqueous, as in fat bituminous earths; near marshes, and standing waters, it is far different in quality and quantity, and prejudicial to health; whence it is no wonder that chymists, in their analysing of dew, should find such different results, that scarcely any two are agreed about them . . . Dew is of a subtle saponaceous nature, capable of supporting vegetables. Some distilled dew has afforded a liquor of distillation, which struck the colors of the rainbow upon glass, so strong as not to be effaced by friction . . . it burnt like spirit of wine. Again some distilled dew having been digested with gentle heat, for eight days, and then rectified six times over, till it was exceedingly subtle, is reported to have broke three glass vessels successively, tho it still remained perfectly insipid. Again some dew is described to be like a yellowish butter, that melts by being rubbed upon the hand, yet grows hard and dry with a moderate heat, being of a fetid odor, and to be found in pretty large lumps in the night . . . The nature of dew, also, differs surprisingly with the different seasons of the year and the various successions of meteors; hence exceedingly small seeds of vegetables, and invisible eggs of minute animals, with numerous other things coming to be digested, fermented, or putrefied therein, it must afford many very different productions by distillation, whence Chemists have formed very odd opinions about it. We can only say that the greatest part of it is water, and that the other parts cannot be ascertained on account of their infinite variety."

The supposed injurious effect of dew was so interesting to Mercurialis that he spoke of it four times: it is excoriating, acc Laitus (q.v.); it may cause vitiligo, acc Seneca; it may cause scabies, acc Seneca; and it may cause lepra, acc Plutarch. By "dew" was meant not only condensed moisture but also exudation from the leaves of plants. If this was irritating to the skin, it is an indication that Mercurialis was cognizant of contact dermatitis, although not so named.

DIA- (Gr through): by means of, with reference to the material of which a pharmacal preparation was made, as in diacarthamum, diacrydium, diaphaenicon, diaprunum, etc., respectively containing, among other things, carthamus (safflower), dacrydium (scammony), dates, and prunes.

DIACARTHAMUM: the mixture contained tragacanth, quince, ginger, dacrydium, turpeth, manna, honey and sugar, as well as saffron, as given by Culpeper.

DIACATHOLICON (fr Gr dia-, q.v., and katholikos, universal): a universal remedy. Culpeper's formula included cassia, tamarind, senna, polypody, violets, fennel, rhubarb, anise seeds, penide (barley sugar, fr Persian panid, sugar), liquorice, and seeds of gourd, citrul (pumpkin), cucumber, and melons, sugar and water, boiled up to make an electuary. "It is a fine, cooling purge for any part of the body, and very gentle; it is usually given in clysters, but may be taken inwardly."

DIACRYDIUM, DIAGRYDIUM (corruption of Dacrydium, a genus of trees and shrubs of yew family, chiefly pines or mountain pines, fr Gr dakry, tear, in ref to gummy exudation): a preparation of scammony, q.v.

DIAGNOSIS (fr Gr dia-, through, and gignoskein, to distinguish): recognition of disease from signs, q.v. and symptoms; a conclusion arrived at through critical perception or scrutiny; cf prognosis.

DIARRHODON: an old name for powders and confections in which roses formed an ingredient, acc Power and Sedgwick.

DIARRHODON ABBATIS: a complex preparation attributed to Haly Abbas, containing, acc Culpeper, sandalwood, tragacanth, gum arabic, ivory, asarbacca, mastic, spikenard, cardamom, liquorice, saffron, aloes, cloves, muscat grapes, anise, fennel, cinnamon, rhubarb, basil, barberry, succory, purslain, the four greater cold seeds (citrul, cucumber, gourd, and melon, acc James), pearl, bone of stag's heart (cervical vertebra of stag, acc Peters; compare "vena iecoralis," which was not a hepatic vein), roses, and camphor, made into a powder. "It cools the violent heat of the heart and stomach, as also of the liver, lungs, and spleen; eases pains in the body, and most infirmities coming to the body by reason of heat," Culpeper said.

DIATESSERON: see tetrapharmicon.

DIGESTION (fr L digerere, to separate, arrange, dissolve, digest): in obs physiology this involved three processes, the first, second, and third concoctions: digestion in the stomach and intestines, change of chyme into blood, and secretion, the "final digestion."

DILL: a European apiacious herb, Anethum graveolens, the anise of Scripture. See anethine oil, and seeds.

DIOSCORIDES (Pedanios Dioskorides), 40-90, a Greek from Anazarba in Cilicia, was a famous surgeon with the Roman army of Nero. His Materia Medica, written about 77, has been described as "the precipitation of all foregoing knowledge of the subject from Plato to Nero." In it he discussed the preparation, storage, genuineness, use, dosage, and effects of simple drugs and described some 600 plants with such accuracy that the French botanist, Tournefort, said in 1700 after visiting the Levant that he could identify many plants previously unknown to him. Few medical works have been so widely distributed. The original Gr edition has never been found; the first in Latin appeared in 1478. Dioscorides described the preparation of mercury from cinnabar and of potash from tartar, gave opium for pain, and used mandragora for anesthesia. (Major.)

DISCUTIENT (fr L discutio, strike asunder, shatter): resolvent, breaking up, dispelling, dissipative; a medicine with such properties.

DISEASE (L morbus, or affectio): Galen's definition was, "Such a preternatural disposition or affection of the parts of the body as primarily and of itself hinders their natural and proper actions," acc James, who said that Galen distinguished diseases of three kinds. The first consisted of intemperature of the similar body parts, and was divided into those with and those without materia: a part may have more or less heat or cold than it ought to have, as when the head is overheated by the sun; or it may be both overhot or overcold and filled with hot or cold humor. The second consisted of irregularities of the organical parts with respect to their number, bulk, configuration, cavities, or situation and connection, as when a part is separated from parts to which it should be connected, or connected when it should be separated. The third, common to both similar and organical parts, were solutions of continuity, such as when a similar or compound part is cut, corroded, bruised, broken, strained, or burnt.

With Hippocrates, Galen distinguished kinds of diseases with respect to motion, to acuteness and chronicity, and to nature and genius, and as to whether they were benign or malignant, and epidemic, endemic, or sporadic.

The causes Galen distinguished as to whether they were external or internal. The external causes were six factors that contribute to the preservation of health when they are well disposed and properly used, but produce a contrary effect if imprudently used or ill disposed: the air, ailments and drink, motion and rest, sleeping and watching (wakefulness), retention and excretion, and the passions.

These external causes are the procatarctic or beginning causes, which are of two kinds, the antecedent and the conjunct. The antecedent were to be discovered by reasoning and consisted for the most part in a peccancy (pathogenicity) of the humors, either when there was a plethora, or plenitude, or a cacochymy, or bad state of the juices.

There might occur four kinds of plenitudes, a sanguineous, bilious, pituitous, or melancholic. The blood might surpass the other humors, but if any other humor were excessive, the case was called a cacochymy rather than a plenitude. A plenitude might exist with respect to the vessels or with respect to strength. The humors might so abound that the arteries and veins contain them with difficulty, or when the strength of the patient fails to support the quantity of the humors, even if that quantity be moderate.

The imperfection of humors, or cacochymy, proceeds from their degenerating, becoming more hot or cold, more dry or moist, more acrid or acid, more sweet or salt than they should be; or by their acquiring adventitious and hurtful qualities which they formerly did not have.

Galen believed that the humoral qualities, acid, saline, acrid, and sweet or bitter, derived from their origins, hot, cold, dry, or moist. When any humor other than blood dominated considerably over the rest, this produced a species of cacochymy because these humors were not so familiar to nature as the blood, or because they corrupted the blood.

The conjunct causes are those which are more closely connected with the disease and more immediately support and maintain it. If present, the disease subsists, if removed, it forthwith ceases. (From James' Preface, pp 67-68.)

How such views could influence medical thought profoundly for fourteen centuries is considered in the Introduction, in the comments of Dr. Adolph Rostenberg, Jr., in particular. See Galen, biographic sketch, indicating that he was a superlative salesman of what presently might appear as organized nonsense.

DISSECTIVE (fr L dis-, apart, and secare, to cut): dissecting, cutting apart, divisive, separating and exposing; a medicine with such properties.

DOSE (Gr dosis, a giving, a dose, from didonai, to give): a measured quantity of a medicine to be taken.

DROPACISM: removal of hair by the pitch plaster, or dropax.

DROPAX (L): a depilatory made of pitch, which adheres to hair so that it may be pulled out.

DROPSY (L hydropisis, Gr ydrops fr ydor, water): mod, accumulation of fluid in serous cavities and/or subcutaneous tissues, usually from cardiovascular, renal, or hepatic failure; cf anasarca.

DUNG: see mouse, and Marcellus.

ECLECTIC SCHOOL: see Athenaeus.

ELATERIUM (L, fr Gr elaterion): the cathartic and diuretic dried juice of the wild, or squirting, cucumber, Ecballium elaterium. Originally elaterion (Gr driving away) meant any purging medicine, in particular one that operates with violence. For purging children, Hippocrates prescribed the milk of a goat or woman who had eaten wild cucumber, acc James.

ELECTUARY (L electuarium, Gr ekleikton, fr ex- out, and leichein, to lick): a medicinal mixture incorporated with honey or syrup to form a pasty mass, cf confection, hiera, and theriac.

ELECTUARY IND: Mercurialis used this; its identification is doubtful. Perhaps it contained Malabar leaf, malabathrum. Culpeper mentioned Indian spikenard and listed "Indian leaf and mace" as ingredients of hiera of colocynth, q.v. Webster (1938) listed four columns of "Indian ---," but not Indian leaf or anything patently associated with "electuary Ind." James wrote of indigo (L indicum): "This juice is brought from both the East and West Indies, made up in different forms. Some physicians have recommended indigo in the quantity of a dram, but others look upon it as a poison, and in Saxony the internal use of it is prohibited." James listed "indicon" as ? pepper or ginger: "Galen said the compilers of catalogues of simples mistook ginger to be root of pepper, whereas they belong to different plants. Dioscorides the Younger said indicon was a plant growing in India, much resembling myrtle berry. Indici potus and indicum medicamentum are mentioned in Hippocrates' De Morbis Mulieribus." In view of Mercurialis' knowledge of both Hippocrates and diseases of women, one may surmise the electuary perhaps contained indigo, q.v.

ELEMENTS: the simple substances or principles, of which, according to the early natural philosophers, the physical universe is composed. Empedocles (Gr philosopher, 504-443 B.C.) maintained that there are four elements, fire, air, water, and earth; and these became recognized as the basis for classification of planets, bodies, herbs, etc. To these correspond respectively the qualities, hot, moist, cold, and dry. Every element has two qualities, one inherent and distinctive, the other derived from the element next in order and, in this particular, its affinity. Fire is hot, and is dry as earth; air is moist, and is hot as fire; water is cold, and is moist as air; earth is dry, and is cold as water. (Webster, 1938.) The twelve signs of the zodiac were associated each with a specific humor and a specific complexion, q.v.; and the complexion determined not only one's character but also one's predisposition to certain diseases and physical weaknesses. The melancholic complexion, or temperament, was related with the melancholic humor, the brain the body origin, earth the dominant element, the qualities cold and dry. The choleric complexion was related with the choleric humor, the heart the body origin, fire the dominant element, the qualities hot and dry. The phlegmatic complexion was related with the phlegmatic humor, the liver the body origin, water the dominant element, the qualities cold and moist. The sanguine complexion was related with the sanguine humor, blood, the stomach the body origin, air the dominant element, the qualities hot and moist. If one imagines that "earth, water, air, and fire" might be translated into "solid, liquid, gas, and energy," it would make more sense now. The ancient ideas are obscure.

EMOLLIENTS (fr L emollire, to soften): are "softening medicines that produce their effects by relaxing the parts which stick together, and loosening them by their gentle heat and agreeable humidity," acc Turner.

EMPEDOCLES, of Akragas, b Agrigentum, ca 504-443 B.C., Gr philosopher and brilliant orator, was founder of the Italian school of medicine, considered by Galen to be on a par with the schools of Cos and Cnidos. "He studied for a time with the Pythagoreans but was expelled for divulging some of their doctrines. He was a poet, philosopher, physician, scientist, and mystic. A skillful physician, he wrought so many cures that many thought him divine, an idea which he by no means discouraged. He claimed supernatural powers and performed mystic rites." (Major.) Not quoted by Mercurialis; see elements.

ENDIVE (L endivia): an annual or biennial herb, Chicorium endiva, with curled leaves used for salads. See chicory.

EPIDERMIS (NL fr Gr epi-, on, upon, and derma, skin): mod, the stratified epithelium that covers the skin and forms the parenchyma of the accessory structures, hairs, nails, and glands, and the cap of a blister when the skin is blistered. Mercurialis did not use the word, but used "in summo" and "in profundo" for the superfices and the deeper part, and quoted Avicenna as having located the materia of pruritus "between the two layers of the skin." He used cutis (skin) for epidermis and caro (flesh) for dermis.

ERETRIAN EARTH (Eretria, city of ancient Greece, on Euboea island): a mineral resembling Cimolean earth, q.v.

EROTIANUS, fl ca 50, was an early commentator on Hippocrates who described the Hippocratic oath as genuine, although this earliest and most impressive declaration of medical ethics is not usually accepted as being of Hippocrates' own writing. (Garrison.)

EUPHORBIUM (L): a brownish, acrid gum resin from Euphorbia

resinifera of Morocco, a cactuslike plant named after Euphorbus (ca 25 B.C., brother of Musa, also a physician), physician to Juba, king of Mauretania. It is violently purgative and emetic. Mod use is in veterinary medicine as a vesicant. Plants of genus Euphorbia are the spurges, q.v. See also tithymal.

EXANTHEMATA (Gr exanthismata): small pustules or eruptions, acc James; mod, acute eruptions accompanying systemic diseases, such as measles or chickenpox. See psydrachium, Book One, Chapter Eleven.

EXCORIATION (fr L excoriare, fr ex-, out, and corium, hide or skin): a tearing into the cutis, a breaking and removal of some epidermis by scratching.

EXCORTICATE (fr L ex-, out, and cortex, bark): strip off the bark or skin, excoriate.

EXCREMENT (L excrementum, from ex-, out, and cerno, separate): that which is separated out, excreted; dross, refuse, waste.

EXSICCATE (fr L ex-siccare, to dry out, drain): make dry, remove fluid from, drain, empty.

EXSICCATIVE: tending to exsiccate; a medicinal agent for drying out, draining dry, or emptying.

FABA (L): bean; see broad-bean.

FAVUS (L, honeycomb): mod the disease, favus, due to a specific ringworm fungus, Achorion schoenleinii, and characterized by peculiar honeycomblike lesions of the scalp and body. The plural, favi, referring to the lesions and frequently used by Mercurialis, is obsolete. See Book One, Chapter Nine.

FENNEL (L foeniculum, diminutive of faenum, hay): perennial European herb cultivated for its aromatic seeds; "a plant aperitive and discussive by means of sweat, which sharpens the sight, and corroborates the stomach, a noble carminative," acc James.

FENUGREEK (fr L faenum Graecum, Greek hay): annual Asiatic herb with aromatic seeds, used in making curry; formerly used externally and in clysters as an emollient, and an excellent ophthalmic, acc James.

FERULA (L) giant fennel, the stalks used for schoolroom discipline; botany (cap): a large genus of Old World plants of carrot family, Ammiaceae, yielding various resins such as galbanum and asafetida.

FESTUS, SEXTUS POMPEIUS, fl ca 175, a Roman grammarian, was author of an abridgment of a work by Verrius Flaccus, De Verborum Significatu, valuable for the information it contains about the Latin language. (Americana.)

FEVERS: the first, second, and third varieties were, as Galen classified them: (1) ephemeral, in the spirits; (2) putrid, in the putrefying humors; and (3) hectic, in the solids (Garrison). Putrid fevers were four: synochal, or continued, in the humor, blood; tertian, in the yellow bile; quotidian, in the plegm; and quartan, in the black bile. "Hectica" (L hecticus, fr Gr hektikos, fr Gr hexis, a habit of body or mind) was a habitual, constitutional condition pertaining to slow waste of tissue as in consumption, acc James, who said it was not mentioned by the ancient Greek and Latin physicians by this name, but that Celsus described "slow fevers," later called hectic fevers, tabid or long-continued, or marasmi. Hippocrates referred to such under the name "phthisis." The eighteenth century meaning was a chronic, mild, intermittent fever inducing a consumption. "Fever of undetermined cause" is roughly the mod signification.

FICINUS, MARSILIO FICINO, ca 1500, was a Renaissance contemporary of Petrarch, who attacked scholasticism. Along with such men as Pomponazzi, della Porta, Weyer, and Pico, Ficino rationalized magic and astrology and opposed witchcraft. (Garrison.)

FINAL CAUSE: see causation.

FLOWERS: choicest parts; a substance in the form of a pure powder, especially when condensed by sublimation, as flowers of sulfur.

FLUX (L fluxus, a flow or flux): the material that flows from the bowels or other parts; an excessive and morbid discharge; a disease characterized by a flux, e.g. dysentery, the bloody flux.

FORMAL CAUSE: see causation.

FRANKINCENSE (OF franc, pure, and encens, incense): a fragrant gum resin from various trees, chiefly East African, of genus Boswellia, valued by ancient peoples for embalming, fumigation, etc.; still the most important incense resin. See thus.

FUMARIA: fumitory, q.v.

FUMITORY (L fumus terra): climbing herbs of genus Fumaria. F. officinalis, formerly used as an antiscorbutic, tonic, alterative, and diuretic, in large doses purges bile and purifies the blood, "hence it is admirably beneficial in all diseases proceeding from bilious and serous humors, such as the leprosy, scab, itch, impetigo, herpes, and, it is said, in the lues venerea itself," acc James.

FUNCTION: see action, Galen's views.

FURFURATION (fr L furfur, bran): a disease with branny scales. See Book One, Chapter Eight.

FURUNCLE (L furunculus, a petty thief, fr L fur, Gr phor, thief): a boil. Mercurialis did not use the word.

GALEN: Greek physician fl second century A.D., b Pergamum in Asia Minor, settled in Rome in 164. His observations, interpretations, and opinions were accepted almost reverentially for fifteen centuries, and Mercurialis quoted and esteemed him as he did Hippocrates.

"Galen's place in science is very high, but his roving disposition undoubtedly did much to develop that cocksure attitude of mind, which made his writings the fountainhead of ready-made theory and 'polypragmatism.' He had an answer ready for every problem, a reason to assign for every phenomenon. He elaborated a system of pathology that combined the humoral ideas of Hippocrates with the Pythagorean theory of the four elements and his own conception of a spirit or 'pneuma' penetrating all the parts. Referring all pathologic phenomena back to these postulates, Galen, with fatal facility and ingenuity, proceeded to explain everything in the light of pure theory, thus substituting a pragmatical system of medical philosophy for the plain notation and interpretation of facts as taught by Hippocrates. The effect of this dogmatism and infallibility upon after-time was appalling; for while Galen's monotheism and piety appealed to the Moslems, his assumption of omniscience was specially adapted to appease the mental indolence and flatter the complacency of those who were swayed entirely by reverence for authority. Up to the time of Vesalius, European medicine was one vast argumentum ad hominem in which everything relating to anatomy and physiology, as well as disease, was referred back to Galen as a final authority, from whom there could be no appeal. After his death, European medicine remained at a dead level for nearly fourteen centuries." (Garrison, History of Medicine, 1929, pp 112-113.)

See disease, elements, fevers.

GALLIC DISEASE: syphilis.

GARLIC (fr AS garleac, fr gar, spear, and leac, leek; L allium): Allium sativum, the European bulbous herb with strong scent, much used for flavoring by the Roman poor. "Garlick is called (by Galen) the Countryman's Treacle . . . accounted a strengthener of the stomach and bowels, an expeller of wind, and very good for the colic," acc James. It "is of an acrid, heating, biting nature, expels wind, disturbs the belly, dries the stomach, excites thirst, causes inflations, will raise blisters on the skin, and dulls the sight, expels flat worms and provokes urine, and there is nothing better for the bite of the viper, or the hemorrhoids." See allium, and ascalonium.

GARUM (L, fr Gr garon): a rich sauce the Romans were fond of, a sauce made of small fish, especially the scomber (Gr skombros), or mackerel, Scomber scombrus. (Webster, 1918.)

GAS: Mercurialis used L aer, sometimes L vapor, but not L spiritus, to express what Eng "gas" now says best, a word coined after Mercurialis' death by the chemist Van Helmont of Brussels (1577-1644) from Gr chaos for a supposed vapor produced from water by cold, acc Webster (1918), where gas is defined as "an aeriform fluid." Webster (1962) used the property of unlimited expansion and the exclusion, not solid or liquid, as the basis of definition.

GEOPONICS (fr geo-, Gr gaia, fr ge, the earth, and ponos, labor): the art or science of cultivating the earth; agriculture.

GERMANDER (fr Gr chamaidrys, ground tree): sp of Teucrium, q.v., esp T. chamaedrys.

GREEN NUTS: probably walnuts; see nuts, green.

GUIDO DE CAULIACO (Guy de Chauliac), 1298-1368, b Chauliac, near Auvergne, took holy orders, ed Toulouse, Montpellier, and Paris, then studied anatomy under Nicolo Bertuccio at

Bologna. He was one of the most learned men of his time. His Cyrurgia (1363) in its many editions was long the standard work on the subject, although it advocated a meddlesome treatment of wounds. He operated for hernia and cataract, hitherto treated largely by charlatans, and used the cautery for fungating cancer and anthrax. With his Capitulum Singulare, he stood out as the only medical historian of consequence between Celsus and Champier. (Major; Britannica.)

GUM (L gummi): a sticky substance, given off by certain trees and plants, that dries into an amorphous, brittle mass soluble in water; or a similar secretion resembling resin, q.v.

GUM ARABIC: gum acacia, usually from Acacia arabica or A. vera, the East Indian variety obtained from Feronia elephantum. "The gum heats and moistens, inspissates, stops the pores of the skin, and blunts the acrimony of medicines. From its soft glutinous quality, it is serviceable against coughs, hoarseness, and disorders of the aspera arteria (trachea)," acc James.

GUM JUPITER: sandarac, q.v.

GUM MASTIC: mastic, q.v.

GUM RESIN: a mixture of gum and resin. Important species include aloes, ammoniac, asafedida, euphorbium, galbanum, myrrh, and scammony.

GUTTA (L): droplike spots or markings; adj, guttate.

HABITUS (L, fr habere, to have, to be in a condition): condition, state, bodily habit, physique; appearance; quality, nature, character, disposition; of constitution, complexion.

HALCYON: see alcyon.

HALY ABBAS (Ali ibn Abbas), d 994, "the Persian sage," was the great physician of the Abbasid Caliphate after Rhazes. His name indicates that he was a Magian, an adherent of Zoroaster, not a magician. His Liber Regius (Royal Book) has been considered the best and most practical medical treatise in Arabic, although it was superseded by Avicenna's Canon. Haly Abbas' system of medicine was the first Arabic medical work to be translated into Latin, a translation completed in 1127. His section on dermatoses was of especial interest—Mercurialis quoted him extensively—for he described skin tumors, smallpox, chickenpox, measles, lepra, pigmentary disorders, scabies, pediculosis, warts, burns, wounds, venomous bites, erysipelas, anthrax (Persian fever), alopecia and alopecia areata, pruritus, pulsatile purple aneurisms of the skin following arterial injury, hemangiomas, elephantiasis, paronychia, leuconychia, and thinness of the nails, tropical ulcer, chronic eczema, miliaria, tinea capitis, kerion, and something resembling atopic or seborrheic dermatitis. (Major; see also Richter, Paul: Über die spezielle Dermatologie des Ali ibn al-Abbas (Haly Abbas) aus dem 10. Jahrhundert unserer Zeitrechnung, Archiv. f. Dermat. u. Syph. 112:849-864, 1912.) See confection, and diarrhodon.

HAMECH: Mercurialis' reference is to the confection of Hamech, a common Arabic name. This individual might have been related to Mesuë Junior, d 1015, who was also known as Johannis fie Mesuë filii Hamech, acc Major. "Hamech (Ahmed) is a controversial name. Some think he is the same as Rhazes, but I am not sure about this," M. A. Haseeb told me.

HAMECH'S CONFECTION: an ancient Arabic preparation of colocynth; see confection.

HARDENING MEDICINES: see indurating.

HART'S TONGUE: phyllitis; same as scolopendrium. See asplenium.

HEAT, NATURAL: necessary in the process of concoction, q.v. Clarification is given in Book One, Chapter Seven, re origin of lice.

HELCYDRION (Gr): "small ulcer or ulcerose pustule," acc James. Book One, Chapter Eleven.

HELLEBORE (L helleborus, Gr Helleboros): (1) plants of genus Helleborus, Eurasian perennial herbs; H. niger, black hellebore, is the Christmas rose; (2) any poisonous herb of genus Veratrum, q.v., esp V. album and V. viride, both called white hellebore. Roots of black h contain laxative; of white, veratrum, containing alkaloids such as veratrine, a sedative and depressant, powerful muscle and nerve poison, and intense local irritant. Stinking hellebore, the louseherb, q.v. "Moses was said to have cured, about 1500 B.C., the daughters of Praetus, King of Argos, of madness by purging them with hellebore, the cathartic quality of which he learned from observing that his goats were always purged after eating this vegetable," acc James.

HERACLES (Herakleides) of Tarantum, 160-110 B.C., was a physician, surgeon, and teacher at Alexandria, so widely known that he was called "The Tarentine." Of the Empiric school, he wrote books on pharmacy, poisons, dietetics, and therapy, and the earliest known treatise on veterinary medicine. (Major.)

HERB (L herba, Gr phorbh, Skr root bhar-, to nourish): a seed plant with a stem that does not develop woody tissue but does develop flowers and seeds; plants often of economic or medicinal value, or used for scent or flavor. (Webster. 1938.)

HERBA BRITTANICA: Lydia Bowen found the following information. "Barton and Castle, (British Flora Medica, London, 1877, p 355) say 'Cochlearia officinalis, scurvy grass (Cruciferae) . . . some imagine that it is the Telephium and Herba Brittanica of the ancients.' Dodoens (A Niewe Herbal, 1545, tranl by Lyte, London, 1578), in his index of Latin names, listed brittanica on p 118; the word does not appear on this page, but the Spoonworte (L cochlearia) is here discussed and said to be like Telephium 'in vertue.' 'Spoonworte is hoate and dry and of a sharp and biting taste.' However, Barton and Castle, p. 404, discuss Tumex hydrolapathum (Polygonaceae), saying that Muntingius, a professor at Gronigen, wrote a treatise to prove this is the brittanica of the ancients. He thought the name came, not from Britain, but from Teutonic brit (to consolidate), tan (tooth) and ica (ejection), signifying power to fasten loose teeth. Linnaeus thought it useful in scorbutic diseases. Barton and Castle say 'the plant has now no acknowledged place in medicine.' Mathiole (p 363) describes Brittanica or Vetonica as with leaves similar to the Parelle (Rumex patients, Polygonaceae, according to De Vries French-English Scientific Dictionary), and astringent, and with small short root." Vetonica, acc James, was the same as betonica, betony, and was also the name of a sp of Caryophyllus.

HERODOTUS, ca 484-425 B.C., the Greek "father of history," was a contemporary of Hippocrates, Socrates, Plato, Sophocles, and Pheidias. He reported that among Egyptians there were specialists for the eyes, the teeth, and other organs, and that Egyptian medicine was so advanced that the Persian kings, Cyrus and Darius, employed Egyptian physicians. (Major.)

HIANTIA (L, fr hio, hiare, to gape, yawn): an opening. Lewis and

Short noted only one classic occurrence of the word, in Q. Septimius Florens Tertullianus; cf Eng hiatus.

HIERA (Gr iera, sacred things, equivalent to L sacra; fr Gr ieros, holy, sacred): "A name formerly given to certain compounds on account of their wonderful or holy properties," acc Power and Sedgwick. Oxford and Webster list only hiera picra, defining it as "sacred bitters" (Gr pikros, bitter); of cascara sagrada, "sacred bark." The word is a noun and means something like "wonder drug" in the recent idiom. The sound in Sanskrit means "gem," in Arabic, "doubt." To surmise any relationship with Eng "yare," fr AS meaning "ready" or "prepared," would be highly speculative.

From Galen's Opera, passages referring to a preparation containing aloes, cinnamon, honey, and milk are cited for "hiera" in the index volume, and from these Dr. Roy F. Butler, Dept. of Classics, Baylor University, provided the following: "Some call the drug the hiera made from aloe, but others, pikra." Galen spoke, too, of certain purges suitable in fevers, the dose depending on the patient, some of them being more readily purged than others, "one of which is the drug made from colocynth, and they customarily call it hiera; but it is prepared variously, that containing hellebore but not scammony being a very good purging medicine." Galen mentioned the hiera of Andromachus, for stomach disorders, as having been helpful in some cases, harmful in others, "as in the case of the hiera prescribed, which those now practicing medicine in Rome nearly all call 'picra,' since the name 'hiera' they consider it proper to confer on (that) made from colocynth. But those who practiced medicine in Rome before us, calling both 'hiera,' for the sake of distinction added to them the one 'made from colocynth,' the other 'made from aloe.' Moreover the hiera made from aloe is prepared in two ways . . ."

We learn from James that Andromachus, (q.v.) contemporary of, and physician to, Nero (b 37, emperor 54-68 A.D.) devised a theriac (q.v.) that contained, among many other things, the novel ingredient, viper's flesh. He did not call it theriac, but referred to it in a poem in Greek as "galene" (serene), "eudios" (calm), and "ilare" (cheerful), words which have in common the significance of Eng "cordial," an invigorating, stimulating preparation, or, in reference to a medicine, food, or drink, anything that comforts, gladdens, exhilarates. Ilare to hilare to hiera, Dr. Butler tells me, is linguistically untenable.

Most of the hieras were treacles, as was the ilare, or hiera, of Andromachus, although some of them were troches. "This theriaca is described by Andromachus himself in some verses dedicated to Nero and inserted by Galen into his treatise, De Theriaca ad Pisonem," James wrote, and "In imitation thereof several other physicians composed antidotes against poisons, which they also called theriakai." James gave the formulas of several. While the Oxford Dictionary derived theriac fr Gr ther, a venomous creature, on the basis of its being an antidote to poisons, especially to the bites of venomous creatures, James thought the preparations were so named because, following the innovation of Andromachus, such compounds contained viper flesh as an ingredient.

Hieras were not indexed by Culpeper, but he listed several of them with his electuaries and confections.

Hiera diacolocynthidos (see "dia-") as given by Culpeper was an electuary containing colocynth, agaric, germander, horehound, lavender, opopanax (all-heal), sagapenum (gum resin of Ferula), parsley seeds, birthwort, pepper, spikenard, cinnamon, myrrh, Indian leaf (Malabar leaf, malabathrum) or mace (fr Myristica fragrans, which yields nutmegs and the coverings thereof, mace), saffron, and honey.

"Hiera picra simple," acc Culpeper, contained cinnamon, aloes, asarabacca, spikenard, mastic, saffron, and honey to make an electuary: "It is an excellent remedy for vicious juices which lie furring the tunicle of the stomach, and such idle fancies and symptoms which the brain suffers thereby." His formula for "hiera picra with agaric" was the same as for hiera picra simple with the addition of agaric and the subtraction of aloes. Hiera picra acc James, who accepted "holy bitters," consisted of cinnamon, zedoary, asarum (asarabacca), lesser cardamom seeds, and saffron, of each 4 drams, cochineal 1 scruple, and aloes 12 ounces; pulverize together, and mix with honey or syrup of violets into an electuary. He said it may also be prepared as a tincture, "tinctura sacra."

"There are larger and more perplex compositions (than hiera picra)," acc James, "as one of Nicolaus Myrepsus (a thirteen century apothecary of Nicea); another of Nicolaus Alexandrinus, which Scribonius Largus in De Compos. Med. ascribes to Pacchius and extols prodigiously for its virtues." (See Pacchius.)

Hiera of iron was mentioned by Mercurialis in the treatment of pediculosis as having been praised by Avicenna (980-1037 A.D.) and Avenzoar (1091-1161 A.D.).

Hiera Rufi (of Rufus) and hiera "Logodionis" were used by Mercurialis in treating alphos and leuce. Rufus of Ephesus was one of the great eclectics who lived during the reign of Trajan (98-117 A.D.). He added many new compounds to the materia medica, including his celebrated hiera, a purgative containing colocynth, acc Osler, quoted by Garrison.

"Logodionis" was used as if "Logodion" were an individual, whom, if he existed, I have been unable to find. "Logadii" was derived fr Gr logas, meaning chosen, acc Power and Sedgwick, who stated that hiera logadii was hiera picra with honey added to it. If an error here may be ascribed to Mercurialis, it should probably be accredited to Aicardius, whose occasional deficiency is exemplified by "tyria," which must have come from Gr phtheir, in the chapter on pediculosis.

The constituents of hiera logadii, acc Culpeper, were colocynth, centaury (knapwort or milkwort), agaric, gum ammoniac (from Ferula), mace, spikenard, squills, diagrydium, senna, bdellium, horehound, cinnamon, all-heal, castor, birthwort, pepper, sagapenum (another Ferula gum resin), saffron, parsley, hellebore, and honey. "It takes away by the roots daily evils coming of melancholy, falling sickness, vertigo, convulsions, megrim, leprosies, but for my part, I should be loth to take it inwardly unless upon desperate occasions, or in clysters. It may well take away diseases by the roots, if it takes away life and all."

Mercurialis, speaking of the treatment of alopecia, said Galen, fl ca 130-200 A.D., praised the hiera of colocynth (presumably of Rufus fl ca 100 A.D.) in pill form and said that "It is best to use this with either hiera of Pacchius or hiera of Archigenes." Since Mercurialis used "aut . . aut" (either, or), the implication is that he referred to three distinct hieras. Pacchius, q.v., died before 37 A.D., and Archigenes, q.v., lived 53-117 A.D. Andromachus flourished ? 50 A.D. Pacchius did not originate his hiera and did not disclose his source. Who borrowed from whom it is difficult to say for sure.

HIPPOCRATES (460?-377 B.C.): The sketch given here should be expanded by referring to any history of medicine text. Hippocrates "was a Greek physician born in Cos. Known as 'Father of Medicine.' Little is known of his life; highly regarded by contemporaries; probably taught medicine at Cos; traditionally but incorrectly credited with Hippocratic oath administered to graduate physicians; author perhaps of some of the 60 or 70 treatises of the Hippocratic Collection, brought together and edited at Alexandria, second to third century A.D." (By permission, from Webster's New Biographical Dictionary 1983 by Merriam-Webster, Inc.)

Histories of medicine by Garrison, Major, and Metler and Metler as well as encyclopedia articles are readily available.

An English text of the Oath of Hippocrates that follows is of especial excellence and beauty. I do not know whom to accredit. The modern woman knows she is a peer and will understand.

"I swear by Apollo, the physician, by Aesculapius, by Hygeia, by Panacea, and by all the gods and goddesses, calling them to witness that according to my ability and judgement I will in every particular keep this, my oath and covenant: to regard him who teaches this art equally with my parents, to share my substance, and, if he be in need, to relieve his necessities; to regard his offspring equally with my brethren; and to teach his art if they shall wish to learn it, without fee or stipulation; to impart a knowledge by precept, by lecture, and by every other mode of instruction to my sons, to the sons of my teacher, and to pupils who are bound by stipulation and oath, according to the law of medicine, but to no other. I will use that regimen which, according to my ability and judgement, shall be for the welfare of the sick, and I will refrain from that which shall be baneful and injurious. If any shall ask of me a drug to produce death, I will not give it. Nor will I suggest such counsel, in like manner I will not give to a woman a destructive pessary. With purity and holiness will I watch closely my life and my art. I will not cut a person who is suffering from a stone, but will give way to those who are practitioners in this work. Into whatever houses I shall enter, I will go to aid the sick, abstaining from every voluntary act of injustice and corruption, and from lasciviousness with women or men—free or slaves. Whatever in the life of men I shall see or hear, in my practice or without my practice, which should not be made public, this will I hold in silence, believing that such things should not be spoken. While I keep this, my oath, inviolate and unbroken, may it be granted to me to enjoy life and my art, forever honored by all men; but should I by transgression violate it, be mine the reverse."

HOMER, fl ca 1000 B.C., the epic poet of Greece, may have himself been a physician. In the Odyssey he accredited the Egyptians with having men more skilled in medicine than any other people. In the Iliad he described 141 wounds involving the head, neck, chest, spine, and bladder, and fractures of the femur, using 150 anatomical terms and indicating the prognosis of certain wounds as well as methods of their treatment. He gave the names of two physicians in the Greek army at Troy who were sons of "the blameless physician of Thessaly," Asklepios, who was evidently a historical rather than the mythologic figure that legend made him. (Major.)

HOP (L lupulus): twining Eurasian vine, cultivated for cones used to give malt liquors a bitter flavor. "The young shoots, or hop-tops, are eaten by many in the spring and are accounted good to cleanse the blood, loosen the belly, and provoke urine. They are good to open obstructions of the liver and spleen, cure the jaundice, and bring down the menses, and are serviceable in hypochondriacal conditions," acc James.

HOT SEEDS: see seeds.

HUMOR (L humor, moisture, fluid): in physiology not yet obs, a fluid or juice of a plant or animal; in obs physiology, one of four fluids, blood, phlegm, choler (yellow bile), and melancholy (black bile) q.v., conceived as entering into the constitution of the body and determining, by their relative proportions, the health and temperament, q.v. See also elements. Culpeper gave a simplistic summary of their influence: "(1) Signs of choler abounding: Leanness of body, costiveness, hollow eyes, anger without a cause, a testy disposition, yellowness of the skin, bitterness in the throat, pricking pains in the head, the pulse swifter and stronger than ordinary, the urine higher coloured, thinner, and brighter, troublesome sleeps, much dreaming of fire, lightning, anger, and fighting. (2) Signs of blood abounding: The veins are bigger (or at least they seem so) and fuller than ordinary; the skin is red, and as it were swollen; pricking pains in the sides, and about the temples, shortness of breath, headache, the pulse great and full, urine high coloured and thick, dreams of blood, &c. (3) Signs of melancholy abounding: Fearfulness without a cause, fearful and foolish imaginations, the skin rough and swarthy, leanness, want of sleep, frightful dreams, sourness in the throat, the pulse very weak, solitariness, thin clear urine, often sighing, &c. (4) Signs of flegm abounding: Sleepiness, dullness, slowness, heaviness, cowardliness, forgetfulness, much spitting, much superfluities at the nose, little appetite to meat and as bad digestion, the skin whiter, colder, and smoother than it was wont to be; the pulse slow and deep; the urine thick and low coloured; dreams of rain, floods, and water, &c."

HYOCYAMUS (fr Gr hys, sow, and kyamos, bean): poisonous Eurasian herb of potato family; H. niger is henbane, leaves of which contain alkaloids hyoscyamine and scopalamine, antispasmodic and sedative.

ICHOR (Gr): thin, serous or sanious fluid from a sore or wound.

IMPETIGO (fr L impeto, assail, attack; L impes, impetis, violence, impetus, force; L petigo, a scab, an eruption, fr petere, fall upon, assail, let fly at): a scabby eruption; mod, a superficial, blistering, coccic infection of the skin, acute and transmissible.

INDICON: indigo, q.v.

INDIGO (L indicum): blue dye of plant source, esp species of Indigofera, obtained by decomposition of indican, a colorless glucoside occurring in the indigo plant, hydrolysed by enzyme or dilute acid to dextrose and indoxyl, the latter yielding indigotin by oxidation. See electuary Ind.

INDURATING (fr L indurare, to make hard; durus, hard): hardening medicines that indurate have "a double manner of operation, either dispersing the more tenuous and dissipable, as in the Schirrus (sclerosing cancer), by their too great heat, or by retaining or coagulating and, as it were, congealing the same, by their over-cold particles, as in the Oedema, they more firmly unite and join the parts together," acc Turner.

INFLUX: a flowing in; see flux.

INFUSION (fr L in-, into, and fundere, to pour): the steeping of a substance in water to extract its water-soluble constituents.

JACOBUS: "concivis meus" (fellow-citizen of mine), whose comment on Galen Mercurialis quoted regarding the relation of dryness to calvities, may have been the Jacobus b Greece 460 who joined his father in Constantinople and became chief physician to Emperor Leo. He was called "Psychrestos" ("The Wet One") by Alexander of Tralles because of his advocacy of the humectant (moistening) diet. (Major.)

JALAP (Sp jalapa, fr Jalapa, a city of Mexico): the purgative root extract of Exogonium purga of the Convolvulaceae. See diacrydium, scammony, turpeth. Mercurialis did not use the word.

JAMES, ROBERT, 1705-1776, physician, matriculated at St. John's College, Oxford, in 1722 and graduated in 1726. His M.D. was granted by the University of Cambridge in 1728, and, after practicing in several other cities, he settled in London. He did not attain a degree higher than L.R.C.P. His "Medical Dictionary" published in 1743, which I have quoted voluminously, is an astonishing compilation with alphabetized Latin titles but without page numbers and with few cross-references, rather unevenly written, with far greater weight in the "A" entries than the subsequent letters of the alphabet.

Medical lexicography became effectively specialized in the eighteenth century in an age when medical historical studies were assiduously cultivated, said Garrison. The principal medical dictionaries in English were those of John Quincy (1719), James (1743), and Robert Hooper (1798).

The dedication of James' Dictionary to Dr. Richard Mead was written by Dr. Samuel Johnson, who also made some contributions to the work, and he wrote the proposals for it, according to "The Dictionary of National Biography," founded in 1882 by George Smith, edited by Sir Leslie Stephen and Sir Sidney Lee, London, Oxford University Press, 1917, v. 10, p 657, the principal source of this sketch. James' articles are well written and contain much information compiled from books, but very little that was original. In essays on gout, rheumatism, and fevers, James' "chief object was to draw attention to his own method of cure, which is praised, without being clearly described. It consisted in the administration of a powder and of a pill for which James took out a patent in 1746. He deposited in the court of chancery a description of the components and method of manufacture of these prescriptions." Of the proprietaries patented in England, taking advantage of the old Statute of Monopolies of 1624, "the most famous were the antimonial fever powder and analeptic pills of Dr. R. James, a physician of solid ability," said Garrison. "It was asserted at the time that both had been learnt from a German named William Schwanberg." The Dictionary of National Biography continues, "and it was clearly proved afterwards that the receipt sworn to in the patent would not produce the powder patented by James and sold by him and by F. Newbery. The chief constituents were phosphate of lime and oxide of antimony . . . and it had a strong diaphoretic action and was frequently prescribed in cases of raised temperature of all kinds, and of inflammatory pain. Goldsmith took a dose of the powder early in the attack of the fever from which he died, and Hawes, the apothecary who attended him, attributed bad results to this dose. Newbery wrote to the papers in defense of his nostrum, and the controversy that arose does not seem to have injured its reputation, for it was prescribed for George III early in his attack of mania in Nov. 1788 . . . The way in which the powder was patented and sold diminished the reputation of James as a physician, but Samuel Johnson never gave up his early friendship for him . . . Johnson says that at Gilbert Walmley's table in Lichfield 'I enjoyed many chearful and instructive hours with companions such as are not often found, with one who has lengthened and one who has gladdened life; with Dr. James, whose skill in physick will long be remembered, and with David Garrick.'" James' "Vindication of the Fever Powder" was printed after his death.

JOHANNITIUS (Junayn ibn Ishaz), 809-873, a Christian of the town of Hira, attended the lectures of Mesuë, Senior, at Jundi-Shapur and became the most celebrated and productive of the translators attached to the college at Baghdad. He translated from Gr to Ar all the works of Galen and Orebasius, the Corpus Hippocraticum, and much of Paullus of Aegina and the Materia Medica of Dioscorides, his style notably fluent and exact. His own works include the earliest systematic treatise on ophthalmology. (Major.)

JOHN THE GRAMMARIAN (Joannes Philoponus), fl ca 500, Gr philosopher of Alexandria, lecturer on language and literature, was notably productive, his works including a biography of Aristotle and commentaries on theology and philosophy. (Britannica.)

JUICE (L succus): moisture, sap, secretion; strength, vigor, energy, nutritive value. "All aliments supply a good chyle when perfectly digested by the assistance of exercise and regularity," James wrote: "It is very little worth their while to consider the different qualities of foods, who use exercise daily sufficient to bring them to the verge of lassitude, who go early at a night to bed, and rise soon in the morning." As to aliments of good juice or bad, acc James, "there is scarce any better juice than milk;" poached eggs are good, the meat of hens and pheasants best, that of geese and ostriches worst. Birds and fishes are generally of good juice, "except such as live in and about marshes, pools, and muddy streams, especially if the water comes through some city, where it receives all the filth of baths, kitchens, and sewers." Sea fishes and quadruped animals, especially swine, are of good juice, the flesh of wild animals better than of tame. Bread, alica, ptisan, beans, and chestnuts are of no ill juice. "Dried figs speedily distributed are of good juice, but retained long in the stomach turn to bad juice and generate lice . . . All aliments of bad juice are not of the same kind, for one sort is cold and phlegmatic, another hot and bilious, and a third atrabilious . . . Meats of bad juice are mutton and goat's flesh because of their acrimony. The flesh of he-goats is worst, next that of rams, and next to this is bull's beef." Among the various foods of bad juice, James listed hare, kidney, testicle, brain, spinal marrow, viscera, fried eggs, old cheese, mushrooms, fenugreek, lentil, tipha (a grain resembling rye), oats, certain fishes, unripe apples and pears, artichokes, cucumbers, and melons. "Of greens, there is none of a good juice; lettuce, endive, and mallow are a mean between good and bad . . . onions, leeks, garlic, radishes, and carrots are of a bad juice, but after two boilings lose their bad quality . . . Thick, fetid, austere wines such as is imported from Bithynia (ancient country NW of Asia Minor, conquered by the Turks in 1298), in large vessels and at a low rate are of bad juice."

KERION (Gr, honeycomb): mod, a circumscribed, boggy, purulent tumor consisting of multiple follicular pustules and cellulitis, due to infection with certain pathogenic fungi.

LABDANUM (L ladanum, fr Ar ladan): fragrant, bitter, dark brown to black oleoresin from sp of Cistus, or rock rose, used in perfume manufacture.

LACTUCA (L): milky-juiced herbs, the lettuces, of family Cichoriaceae, which include chicory and endive.

LAITUS: one of Mercurialis' authorities for the view that dew is injurious, not identified. See dew. Laitus might possibly be a misprint for Laertius.

LAPATHUM (L): sorrel, Rumex acetosa; or any plant having sour juice; see acetosa and sorrel.

LAPIS LAZULI: (L, azure stone, fr Ar lazaward): the hard gemstone characterized by the constituent lazurite, a sodium aluminum silicate containing sulfur; or lazulite, blue spar, a hydrous phosphate of aluminum, iron, and magnesium. If pure, these substances could hardly have pharmacologic effects. Of the latter, even the magnesium fraction is quite insoluble but would be the cheaper.

"Lapis lazuli purges melancholy being taken inwardly; outwardly worn as a jewel it makes men cheerful, fortunate, and rich," acc Culpeper. James described "Lazuli: Cyanus, Lapis Cyanus, Caeruleum nativium, Azure Stone. A hard blue stone with gold and silver colored specks and veins, occurring in two kinds, one that can bear the fire and the other that cannot." The former was from Asia and Africa, the Oriental Stone, the other from Germany and Italy, from gold, silver, and copper mines, softer than the Oriental, the German variety in time turning green. The Asian and African variety was best: "It purges upwards and downwards and is recommended in melancholy affections, quartan agues, apoplexies, and epilepsies." It had a corroding quality with some astringency that Dioscorides and Galen said might be corrected by washing it with water, a view James disputed: "washed or unwashed, it vomits and purges." By calcination the purgative virtue was much lessened. The black stools it produced were due, acc James, "to the color steel and copper medicines communicate to the feces." Seldom used but in confectio Alkermes, a strengthening cordial, it had long since been omitted even from the formula for that. The dose was one dram of the stone reduced to a fine powder.

LARKSPUR: Pediculicide, delphinium; see staphisagria.

LAVACRE (L lavacrum, bath, fr lavare, to wash): obs Eng bath, bathtub, font.

LAVENDER: see stechados.

LENTISCUS (L): the mastic tree, Pistacia lentiscus, or the resin of this tree, mastic, q.v., an aromatic and astringent gum.

LEONELLUS PIUS: the "celebrated octogenarian" who, Mercurialis said, survived pruritus and its treatment; not identified.

LEPRA (L, Gr, fr lepros, scaly, scabby, rough; Gr lepos, scale, husk, rind; Gr lepein, to peel, strip, bark): any of various scaly, rough, itchy diseases; "lepra of the Arabs" was the mod leprosy, while "lepra Graecorum" applied mainly to what is now called psoriasis. "Leper" originally applied to the disease, its victim, "leprous." "Leprosy," the disease name, was derived from L adj leprosus, acc Skeat.

LEVIGATE (L levigare, to make smooth): reduce to fine powder or paste, mix thoroughly, grind smooth.

LITHARGE (L lithargyrus, fr Gr, stone and silver): a fused form of lead monoxide in hard or scaly crystalline masses or flakes. Minium is red lead, Pb_30_4, prepared by oxidizing massicot, which is unfused lead monoxide.

LIVER VEIN: see Vena iecoralis.

LIXIVIATE (fr L lixivium, lye; lixivius, made into lye): to leach, separate by washing, the resultant lixivium usually containing alkali, as lye from ashes.

LOGODION: see hiera logadii.

LOOSENING MEDICINES: see emollients.

LOUSEHERB, LOUSEWORT: stinking hellebore, q.v.; any scrofulariaceous or figwort plant of genus Pedicularis, including wood betony, q.v.

LUCILIUS, JUNIOR, ca 65, was a correspondent of Seneca the Younger. His poem about Mt. Aetna was concerned with volcanic activity but apparently antedated the eruption of 79, during which Pliny the Elder lost his life (Americana). His comment on vitiligo, quoted by Festus, was mentioned by Mercurialis.

LUPINE (L lupinus): fabaceous plants (L faba, bean), of pea family, the fruit a true pod, of genus Lupinus. The seeds, esp of white lupine of Europe, have been used as food from ancient times.

MACULE (L macula, spot, stain, blot): mod, a lesion of the skin not elevated or depressed but different from normal in color or texture.

MADAROSIS (fr Gr madaros, bald): baldness; mod, loss of eyelashes or hair of eyebrows.

MADDER (L rubia): Eurasian herb, Rubia tinctorum, the root a source from antiquity of the dye, alizarin, which produces the Turkey reds and shades of pink, chocolate, etc. with various mordants. "It is both drying and binding, yet not without some opening quality, for it helps the yellow jaundice. . ." acc Culpeper. See rubia.

MAIMONIDES (Musa ibn Maimun), also known as Rabbi Moses, 1135-1208, b Cordoba, was the son of a scholar, Maimun, who was a Talmudist, astronomer, and mathematician. Maimonides was 13 years old when the Almohades captured Cordoba. His family wandered for a time, then moved to Egypt and settled near Cairo. His father died, the family fortunes were lost with a shipwreck, and he took up the practice of medicine to earn a living, becoming physician to Saladin. He achieved greatest fame as a philosopher and religious teacher. His views resembled those of Averroes, of whom he was a pupil, in that he rejected much Rabbinical tradition and endeavored to reconcile faith and reason, arousing thereby the hostility among the orthodox Jews that Averroes aroused among the orthodox Muslims. His Book of Counsel, concerned with diet and personal hygiene, and his Aphorismen Mosis, taken from Galen, were translated from Arabic into Hebrew and Latin and were widely read, and he translated Avicenna's Canon into Hebrew. (Major.)

MALABATHRUM (L): the Malabar leaf, of Cinnamomum malabathrum; also the ointment prepared from it. Malabar, district of Madras, SW India. See electuary Ind.

MALICORUM: pomegranate rind, q.v.

MALLOW (L malva, fr Gr malakos): a plant of genus Malva, esp the common wild mallow of Europe or the dwarf mallow; of marsh mallow. "They are cool and digesting, resist poison, and help corrosions, or gnawing of the bowels," acc Culpeper.

MANNA (L, fr Gr): a grain, or a vegetable juice hardened into granules; manna croup, or groats, the portion of hard wheat not ground by the millstones, a kind of semolina, sizings, or coarse middlings, for puddings or soups; also the sweetish exudate from the European flowering ash, a gentle laxative, containing mannitol. (Webster, 1918.)

MARCELLUS (Empiricus), ca 400, a Gaul from Bordeaux, was the author of a book of remedies compiled from a wide range of indiscriminately selected sources. One of his charms was an ancient Celtic verse, acc Garrison. Mercurialis quoted his recommendation of wolf dung and mountain goat blood for the treatment of lepra.

MARJORAM (L marjorana): any mint of genera Origanum, q.v., or Majorana. Sweet marjoram is fragrant and used for flavoring.

MARSH MALLOW: European perennial herb, Althaea officinalis, the root used as a demulcent; see Althaea. Marshmallow, originally a confection from root of marsh mallow, is now a confection of corn syrup, sugar, starch, and gelatin.

MASTIC: gum or resin of mastic tree, Pistacia lentiscus, an aromatic used also as an ingredient of varnishes and lacquers; see lentiscus.

MATERIA (L): material, matter, stuff of which something is composed, basic element; the first phase of creation, requiring anima, q.v., to give it form and natural heat for bringing this about.

MATERIAL CAUSE: see causation.

MELANCHOLY (L melancholia, fr G melancholia, black bile): the humor, q.v., originating in the brain, its dominant element earth, dominant qualities cold and dry, the associated complexion, q.v., melancholic, i.e. dejected, pensive, unhappy.

MELICERIS (L, fr Gr): honeylike matter in lesions of favus, q.v.

MELILOT (L fr Gr melilotos, honey lotus): plant of genus Melilotus; sweet clover.

MELISSA (L): Old World mints, one sp the commonly cultivated balm.

MEMBER (L membrum): a body part or organ. The word "organ" (L organum) does not appear in Mercurialis' text. Membrum and organum refer to somewhat independent body parts that perform special functions. The modern concept of an organ as a structure consisting of several tissues awaited development of the microscope. The first simple, efficient, compound instruments were made by Anton Leeuwenhoek (1632-1723).

MENTAGRA (L, fr mentum, chin, and Gr agra, something caught; formed after podagra fr Gr pod, foot: gout): "the chin disease," a tetter or lichen involving the chin, apparently transmissible. See Book Two, Chapter Six. Mod impetigo, sycosis, tinea barbae.

MERCURY: see quicksilver.

MESUË, JUNIOR (Masivyah al-Mardini), d 1015, known also as Johannis fie Mesuë filii Hamech, was said to have studied at Baghdad and attended lectures of Avicenna. Attributed to him but not known in the original is a work that was among the first medical books printed and was influential in familiarizing Europe with Arabic pharmacy and materia medica. (Major.)

MESUË, SENIOR (Yuhanna ibn Masawayh), 777-857, a Nestorian Christian b Jundi-Shapur, was physician to four caliphs, the first of whom was Harun al Rashid. He became head of the school at Baghdad, where he proved to be brilliant but irascible, more feared than loved. He was a prolific translator and compiler and also produced original books on many subjects, including dietetics, drugs, fevers, venesection, diseases of women, colic, animals, and alchemy. (Major.)

MITHRIDATE: an antidote or theriac, q.v., named after Mithridates VI (? 132-63 B.C.), King of Pontus in Asia Minor. "The antidote of Mithridates, which was found written with his own hand, consisted of two dry'd walnuts, as many figs, and twenty leaves of rue bruised together, with a grain of salt," acc James, quoting Pliny. Acc Culpeper, it was Gnaeus Pompeius Magnus (Pompey, 106-48 B.C.) who "found in the treasury of Mithridates when he was overthrown, a scroll of his own handwriting, containing a medicine against any poison or infection: Take 2 dry walnuts, and as many good figs, and 20 leaves of rue, bruised and beaten together with 2 or 3 corns of salt and 20 juniper berries, which taken every morning fasting, preserves from danger of poison or infection that day it is taken."

Culpeper elsewhere in his Herbal gave a mithridate formula that contained about 50 ingredients: myrrh, saffron, agaric, ginger, cinnamon, spikenard, frankincense, treacle, mustard seeds, hartwort (birthwort, or melilot), balm of Gilead or oil of nutmegs, schenanth (reed flowers), lavender, costus (annual herb, Saussure lappa, of Kashmir, a sachet perfume), galbanum (gum resin resembling asafetida from Asiatic plants, mostly species of Ferula), turpentine, pepper, castor, hypocist (herb parasitic on roots of Cistus, a genus of rock roses), styrax (S. officinalis yields benzoin), calaminth, opopanax (juice or gum from all-heal, a name for various plants including valerian, mistletoe, woundwort, and yarrow), tobacco or mace, cassia, poley mountain (Teucrium polium, a germander), scordium, carrot seeds, cubebs, troch (?), cypheos (?), bdellium, gum Arabic, parsley seeds, opium, cardamom, fennel, gentian, rose leaves, Cretan dittany, anise seeds, asarabacca (herbs of the birthwort family, Aristolochiaceae, the source of a nonodorous camphorlike substance), orris, valerian, sagapenum (gum resin resembling galbanum from Persian plant, probably Ferula), acacia, bellies of skinks (small lizards, including Scincus officinalis of Egypt and North Africa, the adda), St. John's wort (genus Hypericum), Malaga wine, and clarified honey, made into an electuary.

Of these ingredients, 2 are obscure, "Troch" might refer to alhandal troches. Lydia Bowen tells me, "Trochos is the Greek word for round. Several botanical generic names that begin with 'troch-' have European species, as Trochiscanthes of the Umbelliferae (T. nodiflorus). Trochantha is a section of Gentianus (baldmoney), acc Baillon's Dictionaire. Trochocephalus is Scabiosa. Cypho is the Greek word for bent; no connections are apparent. Cyphi is a perfume mentioned in Mathiole on Dioscorides."

MOSES, RABBI: see Maimonides.

MOUSE (L mus): "The whole animal and its dung are useful in medicine," acc James. "The mouse, cut up alive, and applied, draws out splinters, darts, and arrows, and cures the bites of scorpions, extracting the poison; the ashes cure the involuntary flux of urine; the dung purges infants by stool, is used in clysters, cures an alopecia, absterges scurf from the head, diminishes stones in the kidneys or bladder, and removes a condyloma, verruca, ficus, marisca and the like tumors affecting the anus . . . Of Mus major, the rat, the part used is the dung. Nine pieces swallowed are accounted by some of our good women a singular remedy for a suppression of the menses."

MUST (L mustum, fr mustus, young, new, fresh): expressed juice of grape or other fruit before fermentation; cf sape.

MYRMECIA (Gr myrmekia): "a sort of wart about the size of a lupine, with a broad base, deeply rooted, and very painful. It grows on the palms of the hands or bottoms of the feet," acc James, quoting Celsus.

MYROBALAN (L myrobalanum fr Gr myrobalanos): the dried astringent prune-like fruit containing tannin, from various tropical trees, such as the East Indian emblic, Terminale chebula; the fruit of a palm tree from which a balsam was made, the behen-nut; also the balsam of this tree. "All sp are of a refrigerating, drying, and astringent quality. (They are) beneficial in falling off of the hair and looseness of the teeth, which, however, they turn black. They exhilarate the body and preserve it florid and youthful, render the color of the skin agreeable, and communicate a grateful fragrance to the breath. The chebulic, belleric, and emblic myrobalans purge phlegm; the yellow, yellow bile; and the Indian, black bile, " acc James.

MYRTLE (L myrtus): any shrub of genus Myrtus, esp the European M. communis, which has ovate or lanceolate evergreen leaves and solitary axillary white or rosy flowers followed by black berries, thought by the ancients to be sacred to Venus. The flowers, leaves, and berries have been used in perfumery.

NASTURTIUM (fr L nasus, nose, and tortare, to torment): a kind of cress; plants of the mustard family, Brassicaceae; see brassica. The leaves, used in the spring as a salad herb, are good for the scurvy; bruised or parched and mixed with hog fat they cure the scurf and scabby sores of the head, acc James.

NENUPHAR (Middle L fr Ar naynufar, through Per fr Skr nilotpala, blue lotus fr nila, blue, and utpala, lotus): European white water lily, or yellow water lily, acc Webster (1938).

NICANDER (Nikandros), ca 275 B.C., an Alexandrian physician, poet, and priest of Apollo, was the author of many works in both prose and verse, including books on therapy, prognostics, agriculture, and snakes. Most famous were his medical poems, Theriaca, on poisonous animals including some that were mythical, and Alexipharmica, on poisons and their antidotes. (Major.)

NICOLAUS ALEXANDRINUS: James accredited to an individual of this name a hiera "which Scribonius Largus (De Compos. Med., written ca 45) to Pacchius and extols prodigiously for its virtues." Whether such a person existed is doubtful; whether there was only one Nicolaus, he of Salerno, compiler of a famous Antidotaria, was discussed by Sarton.

NICOLAUS FLORENTINUS (Niccolo Falucci), d ca 1412, one of the masters of the school at Padua, was author of a vast repertory called Sermones Medicinales (1484), which summarized the whole of medieval medicine and teemed with direct quotations from all the known authorities. (Garrison.)

NICOLAUS MYREPSOS ("the Ointment Maker"), ca 1250, b Alexandria, was a Byzantine physician at the court of Nicaea under Joannes III (emperor 1222-1254). He compiled a large collection of pharmaceutical recipes derived from but far more elaborate than, the Antidotium of Nicholas of Salerno, classifying them in 48 groups according to their medical properties; 15 of his formulae, including some for mercurial ointments, were "ad scabiem." An abridged text was published in Latin by the Calabrian physician, Nicholas of Reggio (d 1350), and combined with the Salernitan antidotium into a single alphabetical order containing 1065 recipes. A more complete translation was published in 1549 by Leonhard Fuchs, and this remained the standard pharmacopoeia in Paris until the seventeenth century. (Sarton.)

NIGELLA (L): a genus of herbs, the fennel-flowers; seeds of N. sativa carminativa and used as condiment in Turkey and Egypt; N. damascena, the garden love-in-a-mist.

NUT, GREEN (L nux viride): probably the walnut. Mercurialis used an extract of Nux viride for staining the skin and quoted Tibullus (Latin poet, ca 90 B.C.) as having used it, too. Lydia Bowen provided the following information. "On the basis of our library materials, we cannot give a certain answer as to whether the green nuts of Mercurialis' materia medica were walnuts. They might have been Pistachia vera, from which come commercial pistachio nuts. These green colored kernels, within a red outer shell, yield oil, and they are mentioned in Matthiole on Dioscorides, 1680, p 124, as medicinal. Bailey's Cyclopedia states that this species, indigenous to Asia Minor, was according to Pliny brought to Rome by Vitellius. Callcott's Scriptural Herbal, 1842, states that this species (or P. terebinthus, the turpentine tree) may have produced the Biblical nuts sent with Jacob's sons, although the nut of Solomon's Song is the walnut. P. terebinthus exudes turpentine, which was used medicinally as early as Hippocrates. DeCandolle's Origin of Cultivated Plants, 1959, p 427, says that the walnut (Juglans regia) was cultivated in Roman times; Pliny considered it of Persian origin. Balfour's Plants of the Bible, 1862, p 43, states that the walnut appears to have been one of Solomon's introductions."

"The bark of the walnut tree doth bind and dry very much," acc Culpeper, "and the leaves are much of the same temperature . . . The juice of the green husks boiled with honey is an excellent gargle for sore mouths . . . The kernels being burned are then very astringent and will stay lasks (diarrheas or fluxes) and women's courses (menses), being taken in red wine, and stay the falling of hair and make it fair, being anointed with oil and wine . . . The distilled water of the green husks, before they be half ripe, is of excellent use to cool the heat of green wounds and old ulcers, and heals them, being bathed therewith. The distilled water of the young green leaves in the end of May performs a singular cure on foul running ulcers and sores, to be bathed with wet cloths or spunges applied to them every morning."

Walnuts were included in mithridate, q.v.

"Green walnuts gathered before their shells harden and preserved in sugar, are good for the stomach, boiled in sugar water to the consistence of a syrup. They might be preserved; being taken to the number of 2 or 3 in the evening after food, gently provoke to stool," acc James: "Walnuts bruised, heated, and pressed yield an oil which some use for gangrenes, carbuncles, aegilops (a carbuncle in the corner of the eye next to the nose) and ulcers of the nerves . . .

"The spongy bodies (polyporus, the tinder fungus), growing on oaks and walnut trees are most in use among the barbarians. The ancients used them, among other cauteries. (After shaping them) they set them on the affected place, and kindling them at the top suffer them to burn till they are reduced to ashes and fall off of themselves."

NUTGALL (fr L galla, ? fr Skr glau, ball): hard excrescences of nut shape in plant tissue, particularly oak, due to various parasites, esp gallflies, gall midges, and certain aphids. Many galls contain much tannic acid.

OLEASTER (L): the wild olive tree, acc James and Lewis and Short. Erroneously the wild olive, acc Webster; rather, a common shrub of southern Europe with bitter, olive-shaped fruit.

OLEORESIN: see resin.

OMPHACINUM OLEUM: oil of unripe olive, acc James.

OMPHACIUM (L fr Gr): juice of unripe olives or grapes.

OPERATION: see function, Galen's views.

OPHIASIS (Gr, bald place on the head): a kind of baldness; see Book One, Chapter Four.

ORIBASIUS (Oreibasios), fl ca 325, b Pergamon, ed Alexandria, court physician to the Emperor Julian, who attempted to re-institute pagan worship, was the most famous of all Byzantine physicians. After the death of his patron of a wound received in battle with the Persians, Oribasius was not favored by the Christian successors. In punishment he was turned over to the barbarians (the Goths), among whom he won such esteem that he was eventually recalled. An industrious physician and voluminous writer, his monumental encyclopedia of medicine, of which only a third of the 70 books are extant, preserved the otherwise lost works of many medical authors of antiquity. "His great genius consisted largely in his ability to assemble and extract the really important passages from his predecessors. Living in an age of superstition, magic, and miracles, he steadfastly excluded superstition and magic from his works, writing with a balanced judgment typical of the best Greek tradition," acc Major.

ORIGANUM (L): labiate plants of mint family, the common one the wild marjoram, closely related to sweet marjoram, q.v. "Outwardly it is of frequent use in baths for the head and uterus, and for the whole body under the itch," acc James.

ORPIMENT (L auripigmentum, gold pigment): auripigment, arsenic trioxide As_2O_3, a yellow powder. See realgar.

ORYZA (L, fr Gr): rice; Oryza, a small genus of tropical cereal grasses, O. sativa, the rice.

OXYMEL (L, fr Gr oxmeli, fr oxys, acid, and meli, honey): acid honey, honey and vinegar. "Take of the best honey 4 pounds, clear water and white wine and vinegar of each 2 pounds, boil them in an earthen vessel, taking the scum off with a wooden scummer, til it be come to the consistence of a syrup. It cuts flegm, and it is a good preparative against a vomit," acc Culpeper, who gave formulae for oxymel compound, containing fennel, smallage, parsley, bruscus, asparagus, and anise (compare syrup of five roots); oxymel helleboratum, a complicated mixture; oxymel julianizana, likewise complex; and oxymels of squills simple and compositus. All contained an assortment of the various familiar herbs and were purges. To make oxymel simplex, acc James, "Take two pounds of the best honey, and of white wine vinegar one pint, and boil them over a gentle heat into the consistence of a thin soup."

OXYSACCARA: acid sugar; sugar and vinegar.

PACCHIUS ANTIOCHUS, ca 25, was a disciple of Philenides and died prior to the death in 37 of the Emperor Tiberius. He is known only through the writings of Scribonius Largus, who spoke of him in De Compos. Medicam. The ancients knew the marvellous effects of the hiera with which Pacchius cured the most difficult cases, but he did not disclose its composition during his life. He made a large fortune by the sale of the remedy and directed that after his death the formula be sent in a letter to Tiberius; the Emperor caused copies of it to be placed in all libraries. Several of Pacchius' remedies were copied by Galen, Scribonius Largus, Aetius, and Marcellus. (Smith, 1849, and Eloy, 1778.)

PAPAYA (Sp, fr pawpaw, native name in W. Indies; L carica): large, yellow, pulpy fruit of Carica papaya, containing papain, a strong proteolytic enzyme.

PAPULE (L papula, dim of nipple, fr L papa, the infant's call for food, acc Lewis and Short): mod, a small, elevated, solid lesion of the skin.

PAPYRUS (L): a tall sedge, Cyperus papyrus, native to Egypt, the pith used by ancient Egyptians, Greeks, and Romans to make writing material. Longitudinal strips were crisscrossed in two or three layers, soaked in water, and compressed into a homogenous sheet. This use of papyrus extended from ca 400 B.C. to 400 A.D. See cyperus.

PAULLUS OF AEGINA, 625-690, the last of the great Byzantine physicians, practiced in Alexandria, where he remained after the Arabic invasion and exerted considerable influence on Arabic medicine. He wrote an encyclopedia in seven books, leaning heavily on the older writers, Orebasius, Soranos, and Galen especially, and claiming no originality. He was recognized by the distinguished Arabic authors of this period as one of the most eminent of their Greek masters. (Major.)

PEDICULAR HERBS: the figworts, plants of genus Scrophularia, including species known as louseworts, q.v., and wood betony, q.v.

PEDICULICIDE: larkspur; see staphisagria.

PELLITORY: see perdicium.

PERDICIUM (L): (1) pellitory, an urticaceous plant of genus Parietaria; (2) a southern European asteraceous plant resembling yarrow, the root having been used as an irritant and sialagogue; (3) plants more or less resembling these, such as feverfew, yarrow, and master wort, acc Webster (1938).

PERICALAMITIS (fr Gr peri-, around, and kalamon, reed): adarce, q.v., a remedy for calvities attributed by Galen to Andromachus the Younger.

PERUSINUS: the knight who fetched mentagra back to Italy from Asia during the reign of Tiberius (14-37), acc Pliny, not further identified.

PETER OF ABANO: see Apponensis.

PHALACROCORAX (L, fr Gr phalakros, bald, and korax, crow): coot, or cormorant, the genus Phalacrocorax consisting of the cormorants (fr L corvus, raven, and marinus, sea). Adj cormorant, voracious, ravenous. Coot: birds of rail family, genus Fulica (L, coot, water fowl); also a dull, silly fellow, gull, simpleton. (Webster, 1938.)

PHARUGRON: ferrugo, iron rust; a remedy for tinea recommended by Galen.

PHERECYDES, of Syros (one of the Cyclades, not Syria), fl ca 544 B.C., was described by Artistotle as a writer on mythology rather than a philosopher. Plutarch spoke of him as a theologue. He was a contemporary of Servius Tullius and one of Pythagoras' teachers. He taught the doctrine of immortality of the soul and innovated the use of prose rather than poetry in his explanations. It was a favorite tradition of antiquity that he died of the lousy disease, and this was Mercurialis' reference to him, although there are other accounts of his death. (Smith.)

PHLEGM (L phlegma, fr G, a flame; also L pituita): the humor, q.v., originating in the liver, its dominant element water, dominant qualities cold and moist, the associated complexion (q.v.) phlegmatic, i.e. sluggish, hard to arouse, calm, composed, impassive by nature.

PHYLLITIS: polypodiaceous ferns; see asplenium, and scolopendrium.

PILUS (L): body hair, stiff hair, hair of the pelt as distinguished from capillus, a scalp hair.

PISSELAEUM (fr Gr pissa, pitch, and elaion, oil): pixol, q.v.; hygropissos, acc James, the same as liquid pitch, "prepared of pitch by separation of its watery part, which swims thereon like whey upon milk. It is taken off while the pitch is boiling by spreading over it clean wool which, as soon as it is thoroughly moistened with the ascending vapor, is wrung into a vessel, and this is repeated as long as the pitch is boiling. Effectual for same purposes as tar. A cataplasm prepared with meal of barley restores the hair in alopecia. From Dioscorides."

PIX LIQUIDA (NL, liquid pitch): pine tar.

PIXOL (fr L pix, pitch, and -ol): a mixture of wood tar, green soap, and caustic potash used as an antiseptic, acc Webster (1918).

PLAINTAIN (L plantago, fr planta, the sole, fr shape of the leaves): plants of genus Plantago, common weeds. "A little bit of the root being eaten, instantly stays pains in the head, even to admiration," acc Culpeper.

PLATO, 428-348 B.C., the preeminent Greek philosopher, was a contemporary of Hippocrates, whom he described as a physician from the island of Cos, from the family of the Asklepios. (Major.)

PLINY THE ELDER (Gaius Plinius Secundus), 23-79, author and naturalist, was one of history's busiest accumulators of information. He had books read to him during meals and baths, rebuked his notably literate nephew, Pliny the Younger, for walking, a waste of time, when he might ride instead, and "all time was lost not bestowed upon his studies." In his voluminous writings he mentioned that the Romans used spherical lenses and lenticular burning glasses. His opinion of the immigrant Greek physicians was hostile, for "the Romans got along for 600 years without doctors." His death probably from suffocation occurred at Pompeii during the eruption of Vesuvius. (Major; Britannica.)

PLOTINUS, ca 205-270, Egyptian neoplatonist, studied philosophy at Alexandria, later moved to Rome and opened a school in which teaching was mainly oral. Preeminent among the mystics, he was described as a saintly man who made no enemies and was loved by all, and he exerted a profound influence on Christian thought although he was not a Christian. (Britannica.)

PLUTARCH, ca 46-120, Greek biographer and moralist, was trained in philosophy at Athens. He resided for some time in Rome, where he undertook the education of Hadrian and lectured on philosophy. Trajan gave him consular rank, and Hadrian appointed him procurator of Greece. He died at Chaeronea as a priest of Apollo. Garrison quoted him as having said that Pausanias, a pupil of Empedocles, used fire in checking an epidemic. When Mercurialis recommended burning Venice to stop an epidemic, he barely escaped from the townspeople with his life.

PNEUMATIST: see Athenaeus.

POLLUX, JULIUS, fl ca 150, Greek grammarian and sophist, who taught at Athens, was appointed professor of rhetoric by the Emperor Commodus because, it was said, of his melodious voice. His only surviving work is a Greek dictionary valuable for the information it yields on classical antiquity. (Britannica.)

POLYGONY (L polygonium): herbaceous plants of the buckwheat family, genus Polygonium, the smartweeds, knotweeds, bindweeds, and water peppers; see rumex, and sorrel. "The distilled water of knotgrass is accounted one of the most sovereign remedies to cool all manner of inflammations, hot swellings and imposthumes (corruption of aposteme, abscess), gangrene and fistulous cankers, or foul filthy ulcers, being applied or put into them; but especially for all sorts of ulcers and sores happening in the privy parts of men and women. The juice dropped into the ears cleanses them being foul, and having running matter in them," acc Culpeper.

POLYPODY (L fr Gr polypodion): a plant of genus Polypodium, P. vulgare, the common polypody. Ferns of the family Polypdiaceae have rounded, naked sori, or seed dots, and include aspidium, containing filicin, used to expel intestinal worms. See asplenium.

POLYPORUS: the tinder fungus; see agaric, also under nut.

POMEGRANATE (L granatum, fr L adj granatus, having many seeds): a thick-skinned, several-celled, reddish berry, of orange size, from African and Asiatic tree. The astringent rind of Punica granatum, with many seeds in crimson pulp, has been used in medicine and tanning. "The flowers and the bark are drying and restringent, good for all sorts of fluxes, hemorrhages, and bleedings; they strengthen the gums, fasten loose teeth, help the falling down of the uvula, and cancerous ulcers of the mouth and throat," acc James.

POMEGRANATE RIND (L malicorium fr malus. apple, and corium, bark): an astringent that has been used in tanning.

POMPHOLYX: see tutty.

PORRIGO (L): (1) stretch, spread out, extend; (2) the scurf, dandruff on the head, fr Celsus, Pliny, Q. Horatius Flaccus; on hairy parts, fr Scribonius Largus; of animals, perhaps the mange, fr Juvenal, acc Lewis and Short. Any of various diseases of the scalp leading to scaling and loss of hair, acc Webster (1938). A term formerly applied to spreading lesions, such as tinea capitis, or other diseases of the scalp; p. decalvans, alopecia areata; p. favosa, favus; p. furfurans, tinea tonsurans; p. larvalis, eczema with impetigo of the scalp; p. lupinosa, p. porrigophyta, and p. scutula, favus, acc Dorland. P. contagiosa is impetigo; p. decalvans, alopecia areata; p. favosa or P. lupinosa, favus; p. furfurans, tinea, acc H. Radcliffe-Crocker,

Diseases of the Skin, third edit., Phila., Blakiston's Son & Co., 1908. See Book One, Chapter Eight.

PORTULACA (L): purslane; cap, a genus of succulent herbs that includes rose moss, a garden favorite. "Of singularly good use to cool the heat of urine, venereous dreams, and the like, insomuch that the overfrequent use hereof extinguishes the heat and virtue of natural procreation . . . The herb bruised and applied takes away the redness and inflammation . . . where pushes (boils), wheals, pimples, St. Anthony's fire (erysipelas), and the like break forth," acc Culpeper.

POTION (L potio): a draft or dose of liquid medicine; cf catapotion, a pill.

PREPARATION: the procedure of making the humors ready for purgation, a formal step in a therapeutic regimen.

PRISCIANUS, THEODORUS, ca 400, archiater (chief physician) to the Roman emperor Gratian, wrote on "The Present State of Medicine" in Greek, which he himself translated into Latin. It was drawn mainly from Pliny, Dioscorides, and methodist medical authorities and stressed simple methods of healing. (Major.)

PRIMA MATERIA (L): elemental stuff; see materia, and anima.

PROCATARCTIC (fr Gr, before, and to begin): antecedent, predisposing, exciting or initial, immediately causative. See disease.

PROGNOSIS (fr Gr, to know beforehand): a foretelling of the course of an illness, the outlook of a disease; cf diagnosis.

PROTARCHUS, fl ca 250 B.C., was an Alexandrian of note, a contemporary of Neileus, who devised apparatus for reducing dislocations, and of Ammonius, who designed a lithotrite; he was quoted by Celsus. (Mettler and Mettler.)

PRURITUS (L, fr prurire, to itch): the symptom, itching; the disease pruritus; mod med, itching without lesions other than secondary, such as excoriations. See Book Two, Chapter Three.

PSILOTHER (L psilothrum): an unguent for removing the hair and making the skin smooth, a depilatory; cf Gr psilosis, lit a stripping of the hair, a pellagra-like, chronic, hot-climate disease of Asia and the W. Indies with gastrointestinal ulceration, emaciation, anemia, and depilation. The vine Mercurialis referred to as a psilother was white bryony (q.v.), known as such to Dioscorides, acc James.

PSORA (Gr, itch): the scabby disease, scabies. "A species of itch; see lepra," acc James. See Book Two, Chapter Four.

PSORIASIS (NL fr Gr psoriasis, fr psorian, to have the itch, fr psora, q.v., both L and Gr, the itch, mange, scab, synonymous with scabies): psoriasis, the lepra Graecorum. The word "psoriasis" does not appear in Mercurialis, but Julius Pollux is quoted with reference to Gr "psorzn." "Psoriasis, species of itch affecting the scrotum," acc James.

PSORIC (L psoricus): adj, of or pertaining to psora or itch; noun (L psoricum), a remedy for the itch, acc Webster (1918).

PSYDRACIUM (L, fr Gr psydrakion, a blister): vesiculopustular dermatitis; see Book One, Chapter Eleven. A species of pustule, of which Trallian (Alexander of Tralles) gives the following definition copied from James' 1745 Dictionary. "These are small tubercles of the head, which resemble pustules, and corrode the skin; but the exanthemata are superficial exulcerations of the skin of a reddish color and rough to the touch. Both these disorders, especially when of the moist kind, are cured by an ointment thus prepared: Take of litharge and ceruss (ceruse, white lead, a basic lead carbonate; cerussite, crystalline or massive native lead carbonate), of each 4 ounces, of alum and green leaves of rue, of each 2 ounces, and of vinegar and oil of myrtle q.s. to make an ointment," acc James.

PTISAN (L ptisana, barley water): a decoction of barley with other ingredients; a bland, farinaceous, medicinal drink, or tea. See alica.

PULCHRITUDE (L pulchritudo): beauty, loveliness, grace, health, excellence, comeliness, beauty of form and features; antonym of turpitude.

PULSE (fr L puls, a porridge made of meal; akin to Gr poltos, fr which Eng poultice): the edible seeds of various leguminous crops, such as peas and beans.

PURGE (L purgo): verb, make clean, cleanse, purify, cleanse by stool or vomiting, remove, expel, eliminate; noun, a medicine to purge. Cf spurge.

PUSTULE (L pustula, dim fr L pus, corrupt matter; L putere, to stink, be putrid): mod, a papular lesion that contains pus.

QUICKLIME (L calx viva, live chalk): unslaked lime, calcium oxide.

QUICKSILVER (L argentum vivum, live silver): mercury. Hydrargyrum is NL from Gr hydrargyros, water silver.

QUICK SULFUR: sulfur vivum, horse brimstone; native sulfur.

QUINTUS: see Serenus Samonicus, Quintus.

RABBI MOSES: Maimonides, q.v.

RAPE (L rapum, turnip, or rape): Brassica napus, a cabbagelike herb of the mustard family, widely grown in the Old World as a forage crop for sheep. Its seeds yield rape oil and serve as bird food.

RARIFYING MEDICINES: "are said to operate, for that by their kindly warmth they enlarge the pores of the skin and send forth the humors at the same time which by the said heat they have raised into a sort of steam or vapor," acc Turner.

RAT: see mouse.

REALGAR (fr Ar rahj al-char, powder of the mine): a soft, orange-red sulfide of arsenic, AsS, of resinous luster, used as a pigment and medicine and in pyrotechny. It disintegrates in time when exposed to light into a reddish yellow powder that is a mixture of As_2S_3 and As_2O_3, which is orpiment (q.v.), an oxidation reaction. (Edwin H. Roedder, Ph.D., U.S.G.S.)

RECREMENT (L recrementum, fr cernere, to separate, sift): excrement; a substance secreted from a part of the body and again absorbed by the body; superfluous matter, dross, scoria.

REGIMEN (L regimen, fr regarere, to rule or regulate): a regulated, systematic scheme of diet, conduct, exercise, bathing, etc., for preserving or improving health. ("Regime" here is inelegant.)

REPELLENTS: medicines which "by their cold and binding quality extinguish the heat and impede the flux of humors to the parts, shutting up the ways, and driving back the humor, by which means the tumor or swelling is often lessened," acc Turner.

RESIN (L resina, Ar retina): resins are semisolid or solid, organic substances, chiefly of vegetable origin, amorphous, usually yellowish to brown, transparent or translucent, insoluble in water but soluble in organic solvents, and nonconducting electrically, which soften and melt when heated and burn with a smoky flame, produced as plant exudates, ordinarily not naturally but from incision or injury, and often mixed with oil (oleo-resins) or gum (gum resins). Natural ones of commercial importance include amber, copal, dammer, lac, mastic, rosin, and sandarac. (Webster, 1938.) Synthetic resins, presently more familiar than natural ones, are organic polymers, softer if of lower molecular weight, harder if more completely polymerized.

RHAZES (Abu Bakr Muhammad ibn Zakariya al Razi), ca 841-926, b Ray, near Tehran, a Persian who wrote in Arabic, "was one of the best known and unquestionably the most original figure in Arabic medicine, a great clinician as well as scholar, whose descriptions of disease rank with those of Hippocrates." After a career as a musician, physicist, and alchemist, he began the study of medicine when he was 40 years old, and became chief of the hospital at Baghdad. Unable to endure the sight of poverty and suffering, he gave away such sums that he died in stark poverty himself. His erudition was both broad and deep, and of his 237 works about a half were medical. While based on those of Hippocrates and Galen, his views showed much originality and independence. His Compedium, an encyclopedia of medicine and surgery, is known largely through its Latin translation. His Book to al Mansur was mainly a compilation from Hippocrates, Galen, Orebasius, Aetius, and Paullus of Aegina, indicative of the extent to which Greek medicine had been transmitted to the Arabs. His Treatise on Smallpox and Measles was the first monograph on the subject. Among his short works is an essay on why people prefer charlatans to skilled physicians—the quacks promise cures. He gave the first description of hay fever due to roses. His Diseases in Children led many to consider him the "father of pediatrics." In his Book of the Art on alchemy, he was the first to classify substances as animal, vegetable, and mineral. He was instrumental in introducing to medical practice the use of mercurial ointments. (Major.)

RHUBARB (L rhabarbarum): any plant of genus Rheum; dried roots of R. officinalis and other species yield a purgative and stomachic bitter. "It gently purges choler from the stomach and liver, opens stoppings, withstands the dropsy . . . is usually given in fluxes," acc Culpeper.

ROB: evaporated fruit juice; see sape.

ROOTS: see syrup, of two roots, of five roots.

ROSIN (variant of resin, q.v.): the resin left after distilling off the volatile oil of turpentine.

RUBEFACIENT (fr L ruber, red, and facere, to make): a medicine for making the skin red by irritating it and inciting vasodilation; cf attrahent.

RUBIA (L): madder. The dye from the root was used from ancient times until alizarin, its chief coloring constituent, dihydroxyanthraquinone, Turkey red, was synthesized by Caro et al. in 1869 (Merak Index). See madder.

RUBUS (L): rosaceous, often prickly, shrubs, the brambles, including blackberry and raspberry.

RUE (L ruta): European perennial woody herb, strongly scented, bitter tasting, the volatile oil from the leaves an irritant poison. "This herb, bruised and applied, perfectly heals old sores, Dioscorides saith," and destroys vermin and lice, too, acc Culpeper. It was known as the "herb of grace," from association with the sense of rue, repent. See mithridate.

RUFUS OF EPHESUS (ancient city on the west coast of Asia Minor), fl ca 100, was a great eclectic who lived during the reign of Trajan. While he was an outstanding surgeon and anatomist, his hiera, containing colocynth, became celebrated. He described all known methods of securing hemostasis, recognized the pulse as synchronous with the heartbeat, described the crystalline lens, the membranes of the eye, and the optic chiasm, wrote a lucid and comprehensive treatise on anatomical nomenclature, distinguished motor and sensory nerves, and stressed the functional importance of the nervous system, wrote a book on taking medical case histories, recognized the fact that the Guinea worm disease is contracted through drinking polluted water, and first described erysipelas. (Major.)

RUMEX (L, sorrel): herbs of family Polygonaceae, the sour tasting docks and sorrels; see sorrel, and polygony.

SAFFLOWER: see carthamus; cf saffron.

SAFFRON (fr Ar and Per za'faran): the crocus. Of many sp, the one mainly used in med was Crocus sativus. Saffron was obtained from the flowers, the stamens of which, fiery yellow-red in color, were gathered, were dried in a saffron kiln, and were made into square cakes, the "saffron of the shops." It was, acc James, "a most noble cordial, a strengthener of the heart and vital spirits, resists putrefaction, is good in all kinds of malignant and contagious distempers, fevers, smallpox, measles, opens obstructions of the liver and spleen, helps the jaundice, brings down the catamenia, expedites the birth and expels the secundines. Good in diseases of the lungs and of great service in consumptive weakness. Outwardly applied in poultices, it eases pains and ripens impostumations. Crocus was called by chymists aroma philosophorum, contracted to 'aroph,' sanguis Herculis, rex vegetabilium, and panacea vegetabilis," Cf carthamus, the safflower.

SALIX (L): the willow; shrubs and trees of the family of salicaceous plants; "salicylic" from this stem. "The sap is accounted good for inflamed and bloodshot eyes. The Ancients used to put the branches of the green willow about the beds of those who were sick of fevers to cool and temperate the air. The principal use of the leaves is to restrain venereal diseases. The ashes, as Dioscorides says, are effectual for extirpating warts and corns," acc James.

SALTPETER (L sal petrae, rock salt): niter; potassium nitrate.

SAMBUCINE OIL: oil from the elder tree.

SANDALWOOD (OF sandal, fr ML sandalum, fr Gr santalon, fr Skr candana, akin to Skr candra, shining): the compact, close-grained, fragrant, yellowish heartwood of an Indo-Malayan parasitic tree, Santalum album, much used in ornamental carving and cabinetwork. The oil that makes it fragrant is insect-repellent.

SANDARAC: (1) realgar, q.v.; (2) the sandarac tree, a large pinaceaen of Morocco with hard, durable, fragrant wood known as lignum vitae, thuja, or citronwood; the source of gum jupiter.

SAPE (L sapa): new wine boiled thick or evaporated to consistency of honey; equivalent of rob (Ar rubb, robb; Per rub), dried juice of ripe fruit, obtained by evaporation of juice over a fire, with or without addition of honey or syrup.

SAPORREX: ? sapores. Mercurialis mentioned it twice, recommending its syrup, along with other syrups, in the preparation of the humors in tinea and in melancholic pruritus. A derivation from L sapor, flavor, and L rex, king, is not tenable. Lydia Bowen suggested derivation from L sapo, soap, and Irene Blase pointed out that saporrex and sapores sound much alike. Miss Bowen finds that sapores, the soapwort, is "Saponaria officinalis, of the Caryophyllaceae, a European plant known also as 'bouncing Bet,' with juice that makes lather. Grieve (vol. 2, p 748) says that a decoction cures the itch. Coon (p 198) says that several writers have noted its effectiveness as a treatment for skin diseases." Acc Culpeper, "The country people in divers places do use to bruise the leaves of Sopewort, and lay it to their fingers, hands, or legs when they are cut, to heal them up again. Some make great boast thereof, that it is diuretical to provoke urine, and thereby to expel gravel and the stone in the reins or kidneys, and they no less extol it to perform an absolute cure in the French pox, more than either sarsaparilla, guiacum, or China (chinaroot, Smilax china) can do; which, how true it is, I leave others to judge."

SARCOCOLLA (NL, fr Gr sarx, flesh, and kolla, glue): gummy exudate from sp of Penaea (South African shrubs, order Myrtales) with bittersweet taste and an ancient reputation for healing wounds. "It is said to come from Persia . . . and is put into Trochisci albi Rhazis," acc James.

SARPEDO (fr L sarpo, cut off, trim, prune, clean up): obs purge. Related Eng words: sarp, sharp; sarpe, pruning hook; sarpo, corruption of sapo, soap, acc Webster (1918).

SAVIN OIL (L oleum sabinum): oil of Eurasian evergreen, Juniperus sabina. "It is hot and dry, opening and attenuating, a powerful provocator of the catamenia, causing abortion . . . Very good to destroy worms in children," acc James.

SCAB (fr L scabere, to scratch): mod a crust consisting of dried discharge overlying a sore; a scabby disease, "the scab;" cf scabies, also crust.

SCABIES (L scabere, scratch, scrape fr Gr skapto, to dig; L scabidus, scabby; L scaber, rough, scurfy, scabrous, mangy, itchy; L scabiosus, scurfy, scabby, mangy): a roughness, scurf; a disease, the scab, mange, itch. "The itch; see Lepra," said James (1745), who under "Animalcule" described Bonino's observation of the itch mite. The publication in 1687 of his discovery by Giovan Cosimo Bonomo, an Italian physician 24 years of age at the time, was met with scorn. Johann Ernst Wichmann published his "Aetiologie der Kratze" in 1786, denying the influence of the humors and attributing the disease solely to an external parasite; but acceptance of the true nature of the disease became general only after Renucci's rediscovery of the organism in 1834, acc Reuben Friedman: Scabies—Civil and Military, New York, Froeben Press, 1941. Thus for not much more than 100 years has "the itch" been recognized generally as the disease specifically due to Sarcoptes scabiei var. hominis, Linneus, 1758, although Avenzoar (q.v.) saw the mite 800 years ago. Cases in the United States have become less frequent lately, a fact attributable to the introduction of insecticides shortly before World War II.

SCABIOSA (L): Old World herbs of teasle family, including scabious, horseweed, and daisy fleabane; named as supposed remedy for scabies. (Webster, 1918.)

SCABIOUS: scabiosa, a plant so named, acc James, because the leaves "outwardly are serviceable against the itch, scabby sores, tetters, and other cutaneous distempers, and take black and blue marks out of the skin. They are accounted cordial, alexipharmic, sudorific, and pectoral, good for all distempers of the lungs, as also for sore throats and quinzies."

SCALE (Mid Eng scale, scole, fr Old Norse skal, bowl; fr Teutonic stems of shale and scale, OF écale, cup, husk): scale, as of fish; mod med, an accumulation of epidermal flakes; in metallurgy, formerly pl, the coating of oxide, especially black magnetic iron oxide, on the surface of heated metal, e.g. scales of bronze, copper oxide.

SCAMMONY (L scammonia): bindweed, a twining species of convolvulus; or the resin of the root of Convolvulus scammonia, a drastic cathartic. Mexican scammony, a different plant, Ipomoea orizabensis, yields jalap, q.v. See diacrydium, and turpeth.

SCARIFICATION (fr L scarificare, to scratch): multiple incisions made with scarificator lancet to let blood from small vessels without venesection or to accomplish counterirritation. See cupping glass. Describing the use of the spring-operated scarifier, James wrote, "There are physicians who imagine scarification to be not only useless, but pernicious. The most pure and innocent person, they say, may be in danger of contracting some foul disease by being scarified with an instrument that had not long before been used upon one infected with the lues venerea, leprosy, itch, or other contagious disease; and by this means the infection may be communicated almost in the same way as the small-pox is by inoculation."

SCOLOPENDRIUM (L): Phyllitis, a small genus of polypodiaceous ferns, P. scolopendrium the hart's tongue; distinguish scolopendra, chilopods, including some large centipedes, not meant by Mercurialis. See asplenium.

SCORDIUM (fr Gr skordion, a plant smelling like garlic; Gr skordon, garlic): the water germander, a menthaceous plant of genus Teucrium (q.v.) having a fancied garlic-like odor.

SEBESTEN (Ar, fr Per sapista, having fetid odor): plumlike fruit of an Egyptian, Assyrian, and East Indian boraginaceous tree, Cordia myxa, used in India for pickles and dried as a demulcent. "They moisten, soften, and obtund the acrimony of the humors," said James, "and are principally used in acrid catarrhs, acrid urine, bilious fevers, and obstructions of the belly."

SECUNDUM ARTEM (L): following or in accordance with the art, or in the usual professional manner, abbreviated "s.a."

SEEDS: the "four greater cold seeds," acc James (under "semen"), were citrul, cucumber, gourd, and melon. The "four lesser cold seeds" were succory, endive, lettuce, and purslane. The "four greater hot seeds" were anise, caraway or else dill, cumin, and fennel. The "four smaller hot seeds" were Bishop's weed, amomum, apium, and daucus (wild carrot).

SENNA: see cassia.

SEPIA (L, Gr, cuttlefish): cuttlebone (q.v.) from cuttlefish of genus Sepia with broad body, long lateral fins, and an internal shell. The shell contains calcium, phosphorus, and, in small amounts, other minerals.

SERAPIA (NL): syrups.

SERAPION, ca 220 B.C., was an empirical physician of Alexandria, by some considered the real founder of the school. "He rejected all medical dogmatism, basing his practice on experience and experiment, on the study of clinical cases, and on analogy. His passion for experiments led him to employ many popular and even absurd remedies." (Major.)

SERAPION (Yahya ibn Serabi), d 930, a Syrian physician, "wrote two books in Syriac, taking his material chiefly from Aetius and Paullus of Aegina, also from Alexander of Tralles, acc Campbell. Rhazes often quoted him verbatim." (Major.)

SERENUS SAMONICUS, QUINTUS: a third century A.D. didactic poet. His verses on popular medicine are quoted several times by Mercurialis, that on pediculosis being a fair sample. My translations of his verse that Mercurialis quoted suggest that it may not be immortal.

SIGN (L signum, mark, token, indication): med, a diagnostic, distinctive, objective feature of disease. The contrasting word, symptom, (Gr symptoma, a befalling, a falling together) means a subjective feature.

SILVER SPUME (L spuma, foam): froth of molten silver; impure silver oxide.

SINAPISM (fr Gr sinapismos, the use of a mustard plaster): a plaster or poultice mainly of powdered mustard seed; see attrahent.

SIRLETUS, GUGLIELMO, cardinal, Tridentine scholar, Vatican librarian; b. Guardavalle, Calabria, Italy, 1514; d. Rome, October 7, 1585. After studying at Naples, where he became proficient in Greek, he continued his researches at the Vatican Library. Here he made the acquaintance of Cardinal Marcello Cervino (later Pope Marcellus II), presiding official at the initial phases of the Council of Trent. While remaining at Rome, Sirleto prepared extensive memoranda on many of the important questions discussed at the council. He similarly collaborated with the other cardinal legates, particularly Cardinal Girolamo Seripando, at the later phases of the council. As head of the Vatican Library, he catalogued all its Greek MSS. In 1565 he was made a cardinal; in 1566, bishop of San Marco, Calabria; and in 1568, bishop of his native diocese of Squillace. However, even after his episcopal consecration he almost always resided in Rome. Here he was the central figure in editing the publications decreed by the council; the revised Missal and Breviary, the Roman Catechism, the Corpus Iuris Canonici, and the official texts of the Latin Vulgate and the Greek Septuagint. (L. F. Hartman, Catholic

Encyclopedia for School and Home, McGraw Hill 1965.)

The engraving of Cardinal Sirletus that faces p. 1 of Aicardius' dedication is from the Catholic Encyclopedia cited above, with permission.

SIRUP: see syrup.

SMALLAGE: wild celery (q.v.); see also apium.

SMEGMA (L, a detergent, fr Gr. smegma, soap): caseous sebaceous matter, mod specifically that which accumulates under the preputia.

SOFTENING MEDICINES: see emollients.

SOLATIUM SILVESTRE (solatium, comfort, relief, solace, hence balm?, L silvestris, sylvan, of the woods, wild): obscure. Sylvestrian balm, or balsam? Sylvestrene, fr NL sylvestris, specific name of pine yielding it, a terpene in Swedish and Russian oil of turpentine. Balm: (1) a menthaceous plant of genus Melissa; (2) resinous and aromatic exudation from trees of genus Balsamea, or any balsamic resin, or any fragrant ointment used medicinally; (3) anything that heals or mitigates pain (Webster, 1918). Lydia Bowen finds that "The term may be simply Latin 'solace' plus 'of the forest;' I see no pine implication. According to Dodoens (p 433) the plant solanum (genus Solanum, the night-shades) was called solatrum. Mathiole also mentioned solatrum. Nowhere is 'silvestris' associated with it."

Webster (1938) gives "sylvester, obs, a kind of cochineal." When the insects are killed in stoves, a "silver-gray cochineal" results; might this have been made into something called a solatium?

SORANUS OF EPHESUS, fl ca 98-138, whom Mercurialis mentioned as having gained renown by curing a case of mentagra, was of the methodist school yet was respected by Galen. He was a leading authority on diseases of women, his text on the subject a standard one for 15 centuries. He used the obstetrical chair and performed podalic version. His writings on pediatrics were the finest of antiquity, contained a recognizable account of rickets, and recommended rational precepts as to infant hygiene and nutrition. He wrote the oldest biography of Hippocrates. (Garrison.)

SORB (L sorbum, the fruit; sorbus, the tree): fruit of various European trees of apple family, esp service or rowan tree. "It is reckoned to be very restringent and useful for all kinds of fluxes, but, when ripe, not altogether so binding," acc James.

SORDES (L): dirt, filth, med, the brown foul matter that collects on the lips and teeth in fevers.

SORREL (fr AS sur, sour): plants with sour juice; Rumex acetosa, the common sorrel; see acetosa, polygony, rumex.

SPICA, OIL OF: spike oil, spikenard.

SPIKENARD: nardus Indica, the fragrant oil from Spica nardi, a plant of the valerian family. "Heating, opening, alexipharmic, and good against all contagious distempers and venomous bites, and of great service against stoppage of the womb. It is put in a pretty large quantity into mithridate and Venice treacle," acc James.

SPLEENWORT: polypodiaceous ferns; see asplenium.

SPODIUM (L, dross of metals, slag): the powder residue of combustion; metal or vegetable ash; synonymous with cadmia, acc James, who described several varieties. The best was a Cyprian mineral "of ash color and cineritious;" James mentioned also "a sort which is made of the soot that sticks to the walls and roof of the furnace in the boiling of copper;" and a kind "made by burning the stone pyrites, digged out of a mountain which overlooks the City of Soli" (a Greek city on the north coast of Cyprus, its nearby copper mines famous; a neighboring monastery is dedicated to "Our Lady of the Slag Heaps."

James described the "fossil cadmia of Agricola" as lapis calaminaris, or calamine (q.v.), and gave several preparations of it for both internal and external use. One was Turner's "Cerate," composed of triturated calamine, butter, beeswax, and olive oil, which had "singular properties and good effects in all cutaneous ulcerations and excoriations." While Turner claimed the invention of this cerate, James said, "I have, as I remember, met with it in a very old English chirurgical author.

"The modern cadmia, cadmia fornacum (of the furnaces) of Agricola, tutia of the shops," James continued, "is a recrement of calamine melted with copper and not of copper alone, as was that of the Ancients. The officinal tutty (q.v.) therefore may be defined as a sublimation of calamine from melting copper to the roof of the furnace, where it concretes around iron rods placed there into a solid crust, which is afterwards beat off into pieces like the bark of trees. This is perhaps the same with the tutty of the Arabians," as described by Serapion.

SPUMA MARIS (L, froth of the sea): alcyon, q.v.

SPURGE (fr expurgare, to purge): a plant of genus Euphorbia and related genera, including Tithymalus. See euphorbium and tithymal.

SQUILLS (L scilla, squilla; Gr skilla): bulbous liliaceous plants of southern Europe of genus Scilla; or the Urginea maritima; or, pharm, the bulb of this plant cut in thin slices for use as an expectorant and diuretic, in large doses emetic and purgative. Culpeper said, "Sanius, using no other medicine but vinegar of Squills, lived in perfect health till 117 years of age. It makes the digestion good, a long wind, a clear voice, an acute sight, a good colour, it suffers no offensive thing to remain in the body, neither wind, flegm, choler, melancholy, dung, or urine, but brings them forth. It brings forth filth though it lie in the bones. (It has) an ungrateful and somewhat nauseous taste, excites to vomiting and provokes to stool, is never given in substance but affords matter for the celebrated oxymel scilliticum, so justly commended for dissolving of phlegm," acc James.

STAPHISAGRIA (fr L, Gr staphis, raisin, and Gr agrios, wild): stavesacre, delphinium. The Eurasian larkspur, Delphinium staphisagria, has racemose purple flowers; the seeds contain delphinine, a violent emetic and cathartic, used as a fish poison and insecticide for pediculosis.

STAVESACRE: larkspur; see staphisagria.

STECHADOS (L stoechados): lavender, Lavandula spica, a European mint with small lilac flowers, cultivated for its aromatic oil; other plants of this genus. "Lavender is cordial and cephalic, good for all diseases of the head and nerves, helps convulsions, the palsy, and weakness of the limbs, is good to expel wind from the stomach and bowels," acc James.

STOECHAS: lavender; see stechados.

STRABO, ca 64 B.C.-19, was a Greek geographer and historian who travelled widely, eventually settled in Rome. He wrote on history some 43 books that have been lost; his 17 on geography have been preserved and translated. (Americana.)

SULFUR (L sulfur): Gr theion, same word as neuter of Theiros, the Divine Being, so called "because used in all expiatory and other sacred rites," acc James: "The flame it emits is blue, and the smell of burning sulfur is strong, subtile, acid, and very prejudicial to the lungs." Prefix thio- in mod chemistry indicates sulfur derivation.

SULFUR VIVUM (L, quick sulfur; cf quicksilver): native sulfur, Gr apyron; distinguished from Gr empyromenon, or factitious sulfur prepared by fire, acc James. ("Factitious" means sublimed.)

SYCOSIS (Gr sykosis, fr sykon, fig): mod, pustular folliculitis of the beard. "Celsus tells us it is of two kinds, one hard and round, the other moist and unequal (not round). From the hard ulcer, or sycosis, is discharged a glutenous substance in small quantity and of an ill smell. They both arise in those parts which are covered with hair, but that which is round and callous is generally seated in the beard. The moist kind is for the most part among the hairs of the head," acc James. See Book One, Chapter Eleven.

SYMPTOM: subjective feature of disease; cf sign.

SYNDROME (NL, fr Gr syn-, with, and dromein, to run): a concurrence; med, a group of symptoms and signs occurring together, their recognition serving to identify a morbid process.

SYNESIUS, ca 370-414, b Cyrene of wealthy parents who claimed descent from Spartan kings, was a Greek neoplatonist philosopher of whose writings a number of hymns, essays, letters, speeches, and a book on dreams have been preserved. His Encomium Calvitii was a comic defense of baldness. (Britannica.)

SYPHILIS: Mercurialis used the term, "the Gallic disease." James mentioned the innocent inoculation of "lues venerea" by scarification, q.v. Treponema pallidum was identified as the infective cause of the disease in 1905 by the protozoologist Fritz Schaudinn and the physician Erich Hoffmann.

SYRUP (Mid Eng sirop, syrop; fr Ar sharab, a drink, wine, coffee, syrup, fr shariba, to drink): thick, viscid liquid made from juices of fruits, herbs, etc., boiled with sugar; hence any concentrated, more or less viscid, aqueous solution of sugar, with or without admixture, as the simple syrup of pharmacy, or variously flavored or medicated. "A syrup is a medicine of a liquid body, compounded of decoction, infusion, or juice, with sugar or honey," acc Culpeper, prepared so that they may keep longer and taste better; thus "they have the virtues of the simples they are made of, and are far more convenient for weak people and delicate stomachs."

SYRUP BYZANTINE, SIMPLE: "Take of the juice of the leaves of endive and smallage, of each 2 pounds, of hops and bugloss, of each 1 pound, boil them together and scum them, and to the clarified liquor add 4 pounds of white sugar, to as much of the juices, and with a gentle fire boil it to a syrup," acc Culpeper. The compound syrup contained also red roses, anise seeds, fennel, spikenard, and vinegar. "They both of them open stoppings of the stomach, liver, and spleen, help the rickets in children, cut and bring away tough flegm, and help the yellow jaundice. You may take them with a liquorice stick, or take a spoonful in the morning fasting."

SYRUP OF FIVE ROOTS: An evacuant containing smallage, asparagus, fennel, parsley, and knee-holly (butcher's broom, Ruscus aculeatus, the twigs of which are used for whisk brooms), acc Culpeper.

SYRUP OF TWO ROOTS: an evacuant containing fennel and parsley, acc Culpeper.

TABES (L, fr Gr, to melt): a wasting, or melting, consumptive disease, a plague or pestilence. Specifically syphilitic tabes dorsalis is not implied in Mercurialis.

TAGAUTIUS, JOHANNES (Jean Tagault, of Vimeu in Picardy), d 1545, studied medicine in Paris, receiving his doctorate in 1522. He taught surgery for many years as a member of the Paris faculty, of which he was Dean for a time. He was a scholar with little time for practicing medicine. His book on surgery (1543) was often quoted by Ambrose Paré. It referred to the old authorities with erudition but had little practical value to the barber surgeons of the day. (Major.)

TAMARIND (Ar tamrhindi, Indian date): a tropical caesalpiniaceous tree (cf cassia), the fruit or pod, with acid pulp, used for preserves and made into a cooling, laxative drink.

TEMPERAMENT (L temperamentum, fr temperare, set bounds, keep within limits): a right proportion of things mixed together; the internal constitution, the mixture of constituents with respect to the relative proportions of different qualities. See complexion, and elements.

TERRENE (Eng): earthy.

TETRAPHARMICON (Gr tetra-, four, and pharmakon, drug): a preparation of four pharmacological ingredients, particularly a plaster containing wax, resin, lard, and pitch, used as a depilatory. A diatesseron, also a composition of four ingredients, was similar; see "dia-." The one attributed to Mesuë and used by Avicenna contained gentian, bayberries, myrrh, and birthwort, made into an electuary; adding ivory shavings made it a diapente that was often used for distempers of cattle, acc James.

TEUCRIUM (L fr Gr teukrion, germander): cap, a widely distributed genus of menthaceous plants, the germanders, q.v. "Teucrium heats and dries, cures disorders of the liver and spleen, and is effectual against the bites of serpents," acc James. See scordium.

THAPSIA (fr Gr island, Thapsos): ammiaceous herbs; Thapsia garganica, the deadly carrot, contains an irritant resin that has been used by malingerers to induce erysipelas-like dermatitis. Culpeper condemned it as unfit. James said, "The root only is used, and that very rarely, being accounted of a poisonous nature, working upwards and downwards with great violence."

THEOPHRASTUS, 370-285 B.C., b Eresus in Lesbos, known as the "Father of Botany," was a pupil of Plato and Aristotle and succeeded the latter as head of the Lyceum at Athens. The ninth book of his Enquiry into Plants discussed medicinal properties of herbs, including cinnamon, cassia, cardamom, spikenard, hellebore, madder, and dittany. The root of the male fern he recognized as effective in expelling flat worms. (Major.)

THERIAC, THERIACA (L, fr Gr theriakos, fr Gr therion, diminutive of ther, venomous animal; see hiera): a sovereign remedy, or antidote. Usually in electuary, sometimes troche, form, these complex medicines included mithridate (q.v.), superseded by hiera Andromachus (q.v.). After Andromachus (ca 50 A.D.) they contained viper flesh as well as dozens of herbal simples and aromatics. Galen called garlic "the countryman's theriac." Culpeper, giving a formula for Venice treacle (q.v.), stated that it was beneficial for poison, venom, headaches, apoplexies, the coughing or spitting of blood, kidney stone, fevers, dropsies, leprosies, arthralgias, and melancholy, among other things. James described theriacae Andromachi, caelestis (Eng celestial), diatesseron, Edinensis, Germanorum, and Londonensis.

THUS (L, also tus, frankincense, same as olibanum, fr Ar al-luban): a crude, nearly solid turpentine, called also gum thus and common frankincense, q.v. Thus manna: granular thus; see manna.

THYME (L thymum, Gr thymon): a mint of genus Thymus, the common garden thyme, a pungent aromatic used in seasoning. Thyme oil contains thymol. Acc James, it "is heating and attenuating, good to free the lungs from viscid phlegm, purges phlegm by stool, expels the small worms called tineae from the belly, removes warts," and, Dioscorides said, is a good seasoning for meats.

THYMION: "a carbuncle or tubercle generated in the pudendum, anus, glans, or preputium," acc James: "What they call an acrothymion, Celsus writes, elevates itself above the superfices like a wart, being narrow and slender at the skin but broader above, somewhat hard, and very rough at the top, where it is of the color of the flowers of thyme, whence its name, and easily cleaves and bleeds. It is usually of the size of an Egyptian bean, seldom bigger, sometimes very small. Sometimes only one, sometimes several together, are generated in the palms of the hands or bottoms of the feet; but the worst and most subject to bleed are those which affect the pudenda." Hippocrates said parthenium (matricaria, or feverfew) cures it; Galen applied an extract of figs, acc James.

Thymion means filiform, filiform warts and condylomata.

TINDER FUNGUS: polyporus; see agaric.

TINEA (L, a gnawing worm, bookworm, moth, fr tondeo, shear, clip, crop): mod med, ringworm, an infection of epidermal tissues of the skin by dermatophytic fungi. See Book One, Chapter Ten.

TITHYMAL (L tithymalus, fr Gr tithymalos): any spurge (q.v.), i.e. plants of the Euphorbiaceae, a widely distributed family of herbs, shrubs, or trees having acrid or poisonous, often milky (milk of tithymalus) juice, including several medicinal plants such as those yielding castor oil and croton oil. See euphorbium.

TORMENTIL (L tormentilla, fr tormentum, pain): Potentilla, the cinquefoils. The root of the Eurasian herb, Potentilla tormentilla, strongly astringent, has been used in tanning and dyeing. "Very drying and binding, good for diarrheas and dysenteries," acc James.

TREACLE (fr L theriaca): originally a cure-all electuary antidote; later, specifically molasses. See theriac.

TROCHE (fr Gr trochos, anything round): a rounded medicinal lozenge or tablet intended for dissolving in the mouth rather than being swallowed, as is a pill, bolus, or catapotion.

TROCHISCUS (L, fr Gr trochiskos, small ball, diminutive of Gr trochos, a wheel): tablet, lozenge, troche. See alhandal.

TURPETH: root of tropical convolvulacean Asiatic vine, Ipomoea turpethum, formerly used as a purgative; also called Indian jalap, resembling Mexican jalap; see scammony. "Turbith is a pretty strong cathartic, purging tough serous humors from the remote parts, and thereby helps the dropsy, gout, and rheumatism," acc James.

TURPITUDE (L turpitudo): defect, disfigurement, imperfection; ugliness, antonym of pulchritude, q.v.

TUTTY (L tutia, fr Skr tuttha, blue vitriol): a yellow-brown, amorphous sublimate from flues in copper and zinc smelting, containing crude zinc oxide. Same as pompholyx (Gr, bubble, slag on surface of smelted ore): the impure, bubbly oxides resulting when a metal ore is burned, roasted, or melted. See spodium; cf litharge.

ULCER (L ulcus, any sore or ulcer): mod med, a circumscribed defect involving loss of dermal tissue due to disease, so that on healing a scar is inevitable.

ULTIMATE DIGESTION: see digestion.

VENA COMMUNIS: common ulnar vein, from which basilic arises. (Husted.)

VENA IECORALIS (L, vein of the liver): so called as the vein selected for phlebotomy in liver affections, probably the basilic. More peripheral radicles between ring and fifth fingers were called "liver veins" and preferred by the Arabs, acc Saunders and O'Malley.

VENESECTION: the cutting of a vein for bloodletting. Compare wet cupping.

VENICE TREACLE: see treacle.

VERATRUM: cap, a small genus of coarse herbs of the false hellebores having poisonous rootstocks that contain veratrin; see hellebore, white. "The root of white hellebore, which is the only part used in medicine, purges so violently, both upwards and downwards, that it is rarely used internally, but the black hellebore takes its place. The leaves, roots, stalks or flowers applied to the skin of a living person excoriate the part and produce an exulceration," acc James.

VERBASCUM (L): mullein; cap, a large genus of coarse, widely distributed herbs of the figwort family, most of them of weedy appearance with large, often woolly, leaves. The leaves, "used in fomentations or fumigations, are reckoned a specific against the pains and swelling of the hemorrhoids," acc James.

VERRUCA (L): wart. Mercurialis mentioned acrochordons, thymi, and myrmecia. His *De Morbis Cutaneis* does not contain a chapter on tumors. See p. xxxiii.

VESICANT (fr L vesica, blister): a blistering or vesicatory medicine, which injures epidermal cells so that serum tears them apart or tears them from the dermis; cf attrahent, and cantharides.

VESICLE (L vesicula, diminutive of vesica, blister): a small blister located within or just beneath the epidermis.

VITRIOL (L vitriolum, fr vitreus, vitreous, of glass): a metallic salt, esp a sulfate; of copper, blue; of iron, green; of zinc, white; vitriol of luna, silver nitrate. See chalcanthite, and atramentum sutorium.

VOLATICUS (L adj, winged, flying, fleeting, flighty; L noun, volatica, witch); popular name for a form of lichen; see Book Two, Chapter Six.

WILLIAM THE SURGEON (William of Saliceto, a town near Piacenza in Lombardy), d ca 1280, was the great surgeon of the thirteenth century. He received a liberal education, had battlefield surgical experience, was a cleric, taught medicine at Bologna, wrote a notable *Cyrurgia* completed in 1275. Less rigid and didactic than some of his contemporaries, he gave many illustrative case histories. He described a lithotomy, gave his method of extracting arrows, used the cautery freely. He was renowned as a teacher and was said to have been the first in Bologna to dissect the human body. (Major.)

WOOD BETONY: see betony, and louseherb.

WORMWOOD (L absinthium): European woody herb, Artemisia absinthium, of bitter, slightly aromatic taste, yielding a dark green oil formerly used as a tonic and vermifuge, now used in making absinthe; cf abrotanum.

ZERNA: Ar synonym of lichen acc Mercurialis, Book Two, Chapter Six. "An ulcerated impetigo (Durnaeus, Ruland); we meet also with 'zerna' for lepra or impetigo in writers of the alchymistic strain (Castellus)," acc James.